ALSO FROM ATKINS

The New Atkins for a New You

The New Atkins for a New You Cookbook

The New Atkins for a New You Workbook

THE *NEW* ATKINS
MADE EASY

A FASTER, SIMPLER WAY to SHED WEIGHT
and FEEL GREAT—STARTING TODAY!

COLETTE HEIMOWITZ

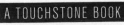
A TOUCHSTONE BOOK
Published by Simon & Schuster
New York   London   Toronto   Sydney   New Delhi

Touchstone
A Division of Simon & Schuster, Inc.
1230 Avenue of the Americas
New York, NY 10020

First Touchstone trade paperback edition December 2013

TOUCHSTONE and colophon are registered trademarks of Simon & Schuster, Inc.

For information about special discounts for bulk purchases, please contact Simon & Schuster Special Sales at 1-866-506-1949 or business@simonandschuster.com.

The Simon & Schuster Speakers Bureau can bring authors to your live event. For more information or to book an event contact the Simon & Schuster Speakers Bureau at 1-866-248-3049 or visit our website at www.simonspeakers.com.

Interior design by Ruth Lee-Mui

Manufactured in the United States of America

10 9 8 7 6 5 4 3 2 1

Library of Congress Cataloging-in-Publication Data

Heimowitz, Colette.
    The new Atkins made easy : a faster, simpler way to shed weight and feel great, starting today! / Colette Heimowitz.
        pages   cm
    "A Touchstone Book."
    Includes index.
    1. Reducing diets—Recipes.   2. Low-carbohydrate diet.   3. Quick and easy cooking.   I. Title.
    RM222.2.H34595   2013
    613.2'5—dc23   2013024457

ISBN 978-1-4767-2995-4
ISBN 978-1-4767-3002-8 (ebook)

Contents

Index of Week-at-a-Glance Meal Plans

Introduction

Many books have been written about the Atkins Diet. And no wonder! The world's most famous diet is famously effective. Year after year, millions of people achieve dramatic results. In more than 110 papers published in peer-reviewed journals, eating the Atkins way has been scientifically proven to produce both sustained weight loss and robust health improvements. No other weight-loss program comes close to this number. Last, but far from least, the Atkins Diet is delicious and nutritious.

We're proud of this record of accomplishment, but as part of our ongoing objective to help people lose weight and keep it off, we're always working to enhance the Atkins experience. That's why we regularly ask Atkins followers for input on how to improve the program. As part of that research, we also speak to would-be dieters about why they haven't tried Atkins yet and what would make them consider doing so.

What have we learned? Some people tell us that the program seems complicated, that they're too busy to cook, or that low-carb cooking seems to require lots of different ingredients. Some aren't sure what Net Carbs are or how to count them. Others don't understand the need for four phases and/or how to move from one to the next. Finally, there's the misconception that Atkins is about eating *no* carbs, which would be hard to sustain and hardly healthy. Ouch! In part, this confusion exists because the experience of doing Atkins is fundamentally different from that of other weight-loss diets.

Nonetheless, we also clearly need to do a better job of communicating what Atkins is, why it works, and which foods you do and don't eat. People want a stripped-down approach that tells them how to do Atkins simply and easily without having to expend a lot of energy thinking about it. The hectic pace of contemporary life, compounded by the need to juggle work and family responsibilities, means most people have less time than ever to plan meals, shop, cook, and track their food intake.

Therein lies the purpose (and the heart) of *The New Atkins Made Easy*: to make the program easier than ever before, both to understand and to follow. And that begins with how to get started—today. Getting meals on the table faster and easier is central to this objective. You should be able to pick up this book, head right out to the grocery store for a few quick supplies, and start your transformation the same day. No muss, no fuss—just rapid results. The Atkins line of low-carb foods, including frozen meals as well as bars and shakes, also makes it easier than ever to do Atkins.

EASY TO UNDERSTAND

The basic principles upon which Atkins is based are surprisingly simple, as are the steps you follow to achieve results. In a nutshell, here's how Atkins works:

- You eat a bit more protein—think chicken, fish, shellfish, pork, beef, and tofu; more olive oil, butter, avocado, and other delectable fats that give food flavor; and lots of leafy greens and other vegetables.

- You initially hold off on higher-carb vegetables, as well as fruit and whole grains.
- You omit starchy, sugary carbohydrate foods low in nutrients, such as bagels and sweetened breakfast cereals.

With these few simple changes your body burns its own fat for energy, while suppressing your appetite and eliminating cravings. The result? You lose the fat on your tummy, tush, hips, and elsewhere, all without undue hunger.

The power of Atkins is based on this remarkable but simple process that shifts your body from burning primarily carbohydrates for energy to burning primarily fat. In Chapter 1, we'll explore how you can quickly and easily make your metabolism work with you rather than resist you at every turn.

EASY TO DO

With this book in hand along with a supply of delicious Atkins bars, shakes, low-carb foods, and frozen meals, you'll have all the tools you'll need to get going on your weight-loss journey, including:

- Step-by-step visuals that show which foods to add back when, to help simplify the path to success
- Simplified meal plans for breakfast, lunch, dinner, and snacks, using everyday pantry items and complete with shopping lists
- Easy and tasty low-carb recipes that use a minimum of ingredients

You'll also learn how to:

- Shop the supermarket for Atkins-friendly options—more appear every day, including a great line of our own Atkins frozen meals

- Modify family meals to make them Atkins friendly
- Put together a delicious low-carb menu without breaking the bank
- Maneuver through the maze of eating away from home by identifying which foods you can eat in different kinds of restaurants, as well as in fast-food places, and even at food carts
- Prepare a strategy—ahead of time—to help stop a binge in its tracks
- Get the most out of your digital or printed food journal
- Use online resources and mobile apps such as the Atkins Carb Counter and Acceptable Foods Lists and customized meal plans

ATKINS YOUR WAY

Another way in which we've made Atkins easier is by enabling you to customize it to your needs and the responses of your body. For example, you may prefer to lose most of your weight in the first phase of the program. Or you may choose instead to move quickly through the first phase, begin to introduce greater food variety, and lose most of your weight in the second phase. The trade-off may be slightly slower weight loss. Decide which one works better for you, and then follow the road map for that path. Whether you opt for the Fast Track or the Slow and Steady approach, you'll find all the details you need to succeed in the following chapters.

With these added features, you'll find it easy to achieve your weight-loss goal. How can I be so sure? Because I've seen it work for thousands of people just like you. I know that every weight-loss program makes such promises. But in this case the evidence is undeniable. You could lose up to 15 pounds in the first two weeks. (Obviously, results vary based on your body type, lifestyle, and other factors.) Yes, that's right, about a pound a day! It's a simple, delectable way of eating you can follow not just for a few weeks, but also for the rest of your life.

HOW ATKINS IS DIFFERENT

I'm not the only one singing the praises of the Atkins Diet. Millions of people around the world have opted for this program and have an impressive track record of success. Here's how Atkins is different from other leading diets:

- *You'll see results quickly.* After just a few days, your clothes will begin to fit better. Talk about motivation!
- *You're never hungry.* Even as you cut down on carbohydrates (or carbs, as we usually refer to them), you eat every few hours. Three meals and two snacks a day mean no torturous between-meal tummy rumbling and no uncontrollable appetite at the next meal.
- *The food is delicious.* The quality and variety of food on Atkins is truly unparalleled. There's no way you'll stay with any dietary plan—no matter what the promised benefits—for more than a few weeks if the food is tasteless and you're restricted to minuscule portions. Where else can you have a cheese omelet with a side of salsa for breakfast, a chef salad topped with grilled chicken and blue cheese dressing for lunch, and broiled salmon with creamed spinach and sliced tomatoes for dinner? And then there are two yummy snacks, perhaps half an avocado in the morning and a chocolate shake midafternoon. Believe it or not, even with all this food you'll still lose weight!
- *You don't have to exercise to lose weight.* Though it's a good idea for other reasons, you don't *have* to engage in physical activity to get the benefits of the Atkins Diet.
- *Fat is not forbidden.* Eliminate empty carbs, and there's no problem eating healthful fats such as olive oil, avocados, high-oleic safflower oil, and flaxseed oil. Amazing but true: the fat you eat actually helps you burn the fat on your body.

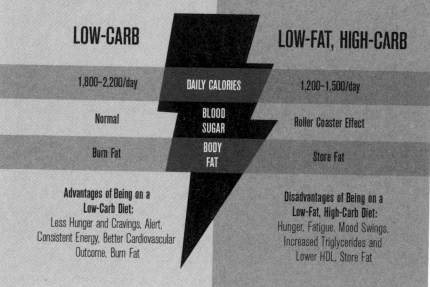

ADVANTAGES OF EATING LOW CARB

LOW-CARB		LOW-FAT, HIGH-CARB
1,800–2,200/day	DAILY CALORIES	1,200–1,500/day
Normal	BLOOD SUGAR	Roller Coaster Effect
Burn Fat	BODY FAT	Store Fat
Advantages of Being on a Low-Carb Diet: Less Hunger and Cravings, Alert, Consistent Energy, Better Cardiovascular Outcome, Burn Fat		Disadvantages of Being on a Low-Fat, High-Carb Diet: Hunger, Fatigue, Mood Swings, Increased Triglycerides and Lower HDL, Store Fat

- *It's affordable.* Poultry, eggs, burgers, and other inexpensive items are perfectly acceptable sources of protein. If you wish, confine your protein choices to fish or even vegetable sources of protein. The Atkins program is incredibly flexible.
- *You'll still eat plenty of veggies.* While you'll ditch starchy and sugary processed foods, Atkins is not and never has been about *no* carbs. Atkins recommends a minimum of six servings of vegetables a day (and, depending on which veggies you choose, you might actually get up to twelve servings). This exceeds the U.S. Department of Agriculture (USDA) dietary guidelines. Those veggies will also give you lots of health-promoting fiber, antioxidants, and more.
- *It's easy to stick with Atkins.* The process of gradually reintroducing carbohydrate foods while continuing to shed pounds (and, later, maintaining weight loss) is the key to lasting success with

Atkins. It's why so many people consider themselves "Atkins loy-
alists" who have made the program part of their lifestyle.

- *Atkins is good for your health.* Study after study shows that eating
  a low-carb diet improves your cholesterol profile and blood sugar
  levels, as well as other health markers. Following a low-carb
  lifestyle can also reverse metabolic syndrome and even type 2
  diabetes.

ABOUT ME

I spent the first ten years of my nutrition career counseling thousands of patients in doctors' offices in the New York City area on diet
and lifestyle changes. In my next twenty years as a nutritionist I've
been employed in one capacity or another by Atkins. For five years at
the Atkins Center I worked one-on-one with thousands of patients
to help them slim down and deal with health problems. In the next
fifteen years at Atkins Nutritionals, I've observed and advised many
thousands of members of the Atkins Community online in their
weight control efforts. I think it's fair to say that when it comes to
eating habits and weight reduction, I've seen and heard it all. Now I'm
excited at the opportunity to be your coach as you transform yourself into the new you. And, as always, you can communicate with me
through my blog on atkins.com.

LET'S GET STARTED

If you're new to Atkins, welcome aboard. And if this is not the first
time you've embarked on the program, I promise that you'll find it
easier than before. In either case, I'll repeat my original promise: try
Atkins and you *will* lose weight.

All you have to lose are those pesky extra pounds. But what you
have to gain is huge: for starters, a slimmer figure, renewed energy,
confidence, a sense of being in control, and self-respect—and maybe

even a whole new wardrobe. Plus stay with Atkins once you banish your extra pounds and you'll enjoy *permanent* weight control and enhanced health. Your new way of eating will let the new you emerge!

Remember, I'll be with you every step of the way. Now turn the page and let's get down to business.

PART I

WHAT YOU NEED TO KNOW

CHAPTER 1

HOW ATKINS WORKS

Now that you know how easy, effective, and delicious Atkins is, I'm sure you're eager to get going ASAP, but hold your horses for just a moment. To get fabulous results and get them fast, you need to understand a few basics about how your body turns food into energy—the process called metabolism—and how that impacts weight loss. Some of that energy is used immediately, and the rest is stored. Whether you're brushing your teeth or running to catch a bus, your body draws on that stored energy. In addition to these conscious actions, countless other functions, including breathing, pumping blood through your body, digestion, and powering your brain cells, also call on your energy stores.

Carbohydrate and fat are the body's two sources of fuel. A low-fat diet is inevitably high in carbs, and when you take in more carbs than your body needs, it stores excess carbs as fat. Yes, sugar and other carbs convert to fat! That's one reason it's so hard to lose weight and keep it off on a low-fat diet. You have to cut way back on calories or you'll never burn your body fat. As a result, you're famished much of the time, and not many people can tolerate that for long. If you've tried low-fat weight-loss diets in the past, you know exactly what I'm talking about.

However, if you restrict carbs sufficiently, as you do on Atkins, your body switches to its backup fuel, fat. Doing Atkins rebalances the ratio of fat to carbohydrate, transforming your metabolism from one that *stores* fat to one that *burns* fat. And when you're burning both dietary and body fat, you lose weight. That's the Atkins paradox: you can eat more fat, but that doesn't make you fat. In fact, as long as you control your carb intake, eating delicious fatty foods such as avocado and olive oil enables you to slim down. And once you reach a good weight for your height, build, and age, this metabolic shift will continue to keep you slim. But the good news doesn't end there: burning fat can also usually stop metabolic syndrome, aka prediabetes, in its tracks, and can even reverse type 2 diabetes.

IGNITE YOUR FAT-BURNING ENGINE

To understand how shifting to a fat metabolism results in weight loss, it helps to compare your body to a hybrid car. When the electricity stored in the engine battery is used up, the car automatically switches over to burning gasoline. Likewise, your body always burns carbs before fat for energy. But when the carbs (in the form of blood sugar) are used up, your body switches over to burning fat for energy. This dual-fuel metabolism enabled our ancient ancestors to survive when food was scarce. But today, because most of us eat too much—or at least too many carbs—there's rarely or never a need to use our backup fuel.

So how do you help your body make the switch? Significantly cut back on your carb intake, and bingo—your fat metabolism kicks in. This is the essence of the Atkins Diet: control carbs to burn fat. If this sounds like hocus-pocus, remember that a large and ever-growing body of scientific research supports not just the efficacy of the low-carb approach, but also its safety. For more on the fat-burning metabolism and the research that supports it, see the Afterword, written by Jeff S. Volek, Ph.D., R.D., on page 297.

THE EFFECTS OF EATING A HIGH-CARB DIET

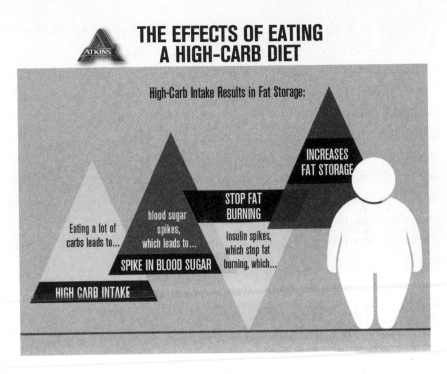

High-Carb Intake Results in Fat Storage:

INCREASES FAT STORAGE

STOP FAT BURNING

blood sugar spikes, which leads to...

Eating a lot of carbs leads to...

insulin spikes, which stop fat burning, which...

SPIKE IN BLOOD SUGAR

HIGH CARB INTAKE

THE EFFECTS OF EATING A LOW-CARB DIET

Low-Carb Intake Increases Fat Burning:

LOW-CARB INTAKE

NORMAL BLOOD SUGAR

Eating a low-carb diet leads to...

normal insulin levels, so your body can burn fat, which...

normal blood sugar levels, which leads to...

SHRINKS FAT CELLS

INCREASES FAT BURNING

GET OFF THE BLOOD SUGAR ROLLER COASTER

Have you ever eaten a high-carb meal—think about Thanksgiving dinner—only to find yourself craving another slice of pumpkin pie topped with vanilla ice cream a few hours later? Or maybe you chow down on a breakfast of cold cereal (often containing a lot of added sugar) and milk (full of natural sugar), a glass of OJ (liquid sugar), and a cup of coffee or tea with a few more teaspoons of sugar. This high-carb trifecta quickly boosts your blood sugar level, stimulating the release of insulin to transport the sugar to your body's cells. This perfectly normal process keeps your blood sugar level within a safe range.

If you're young, fit, and have no predisposition to blood sugar issues, you may be able to get away with eating this way for years. (Or not—sad to say, more and more children are developing high blood sugar and even type 2 diabetes.) If insulin overcompensates, after a couple of hours your blood sugar level drops quickly and precipitously. You feel sleepy, jittery, or unable to concentrate. Your body's response to this energy drain is to crave another high-sugar, high-starch, energy-boosting meal or snack. Welcome to the blood sugar roller coaster.

So you give in and have another sweetened cup of coffee or tea to rev up your engine, perhaps accompanied by a doughnut or muffin. And the process starts all over again! You can see why I compare these rapid shifts between energy highs and lows to a roller-coaster ride. But getting off the roller coaster is easy—and I suspect you already know how. By controlling your carb intake and eating high-fiber carb foods with proteins and fats, you smooth out the wild swings and keep your blood sugar on an even keel. By minimizing periods of low blood sugar, which triggers hunger for all the wrong foods, you'll find it easy to stay in control and not overeat. And, thanks to this newfound sense of control, you begin to shed pounds. That's why Atkins is so effective.

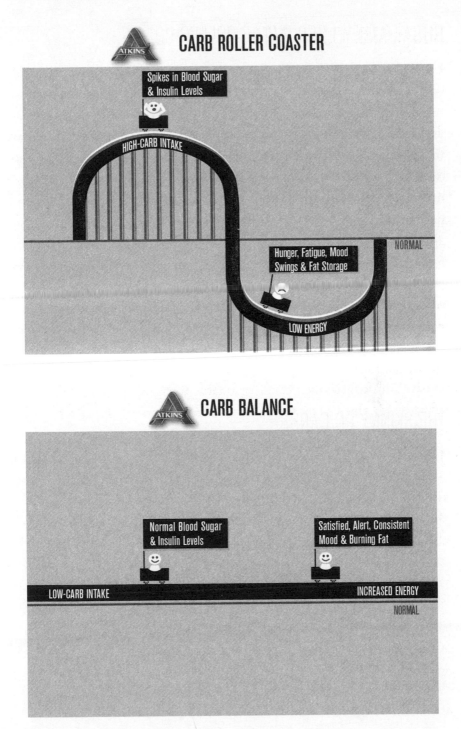

SUGAR AND YOUR HEALTH

Eating processed foods full of sugar hurts you in two ways. First, obviously, you're adding empty carbs to your diet. And you're probably also not eating enough foods full of the vitamins, minerals, antioxidants, and fiber that help keep you healthy. We've long known that sugar intake promotes tooth decay and obesity, but study after study also directly links the intake of excess sugar to an increased risk for cancer, diabetes, gastrointestinal problems, eye diseases, osteoporosis, coronary heart disease, and other inflammatory diseases. Excess sugar also appears to affect the brain and has been implicated in poor memory formation, learning disabilities, depression, and even dementia. As you zero in on your goal weight, reducing your risk for all these conditions is also a powerful motivator for continuing to avoid added sugar whenever possible. Sidebars throughout this book detail the dangers of added sugar in all its forms and point out where it lurks and what to substitute for it.

THE SKINNY ON CARBS

You know fat when you see it. Butter? Check. Olive oil? Check. Ditto with protein, although animal protein such as chicken, salmon, and the like may spring to mind before lentils, tofu, and other vegetable sources. But I suspect some of you may be scratching your head and saying, "So what are carbs anyway?" Here's what you need to know:

- Carbs are found in all plant foods, including grains, cereals, potatoes, bread, and pasta. And everyone knows that sugar, which comes from plants, is packed with carbs. But *all* vegetables, from arugula to zucchini, and *all* fruits are also carb foods.
- Carb counts of different foods vary enormously. Berries are relatively low in carbs, for example, while bananas are at the other end of the spectrum. Likewise, salad greens barely register on

the carb scale, but potatoes and other starchy veggies such as sweet peas are much higher in carbs.

- Lettuce, spinach, and other leafy greens, along with dozens of other low-carb vegetables—we call them "foundation vegetables" to distinguish them from starchy vegetables—make up most of your initial carb intake on the Atkins Diet. (See page 38 for more details.)
- The amount of carbs (as well as of protein and fat) in any food is measured in grams.
- Usually the higher the number of grams of carbs per serving, the faster and greater the impact on your blood sugar.
- Removing the fiber from food, as is the case in most fruit juice and in white flour and other refined grain products, effectively raises the impact on blood sugar. It's preferable to eat whole fruit and brown rice and other whole grains.
- Dairy products also contain some carbs, in the form of milk sugars.
- Carbs show up in a few shellfish as well, although not in finned fish. (See page 35 for more on shellfish.)

THE CORE CARBS

It's important to understand that Atkins is not about eliminating all carbs. But there are *some* carb foods you'll avoid and others you'll eliminate initially. Early in the program, you'll focus on certain foods, which will continue to be the core of the New Atkins Diet as you increase and broaden your carb intake over time. The quality of the carbs you eat is as important as the quantity. Initially, you'll significantly lower your carb intake and you'll eat primarily whole-food carbohydrates, including as many non-starchy vegetables as possible. You can also have most Atkins snacks, shakes, and treats, as well as the new line of Atkins frozen meals. As you get closer to your goal weight, you'll reintroduce other high-fiber carbs, in a certain order, following the Carb Ladder (page 14).

THE SCOOP ON SUGAR: FAT TOOK THE HIT FOR SUGAR

For decades, fat was considered the main culprit in the obesity epidemic. We ate low-fat cookies and drank skim milk, but our collective waistline continued to expand. The real culprit, sugar, was hiding in plain sight in many so-called healthful foods and beverages. But today more and more nutritionists and doctors have called out sugar as a major cause of the obesity epidemic—something we at Atkins have been saying for decades. The typical American now eats a staggering 116 pounds of added sugars (including table sugar, high-fructose corn syrup, and other caloric sweeteners) a year. And that's on top of the naturally occurring sugar we consume in fruits, vegetables, grains, dairy products, and other foods.

THE IMPORTANCE OF PROTEIN

Protein contains the amino acids that are the building blocks from which your body preserves existing (and forms new) muscle tissue, flesh, and nerves. Among the other functions enabled by this protein powerhouse are:

- Keeping warm
- Blood clotting
- Healthy brain function
- Manufacturing hormones, enzymes, and antibodies
- Maintaining an alkali/acid balance

Eating an optimal amount of protein (and fat) while cutting down on carbs accomplishes a number of things, including:

- Satiating you, so you feel pleasantly full
- Moderating your blood sugar level, helping tame your appetite for several hours
- Protecting muscle, so you shed only fat pounds once you've eliminated excess fluid in the first few days of the program

In no way is Atkins a high-protein diet. Guidelines call for 4–6 ounces (cooked weight) of protein foods at each meal. A petite, desk-bound woman might be satisfied with 4 ounces, while an active guy might aim for 6 ounces. (A very big guy might even want 8 ounces.) But you won't have to weigh protein servings. Just compare them to certain common objects and pretty soon you'll be able to eyeball protein and other food portions accurately. (See "Portion Control" on page 58.) Your daily intake of protein foods will range between 12 and 18 ounces (cooked weight) a day.

DIETARY FAT MAKES ATKINS WORK

That leaves us with the third, last, and most (unfairly) maligned macronutrient: fat, which often comes packaged with protein in foods. Okay, I know what you're thinking: "Why can't I just eat no fat or very little fat and burn only my body fat?" There are several reasons this approach won't work:

- Eating adequate fat (at least healthy fats) is essential for life.
- Dietary fats allow your body to absorb the fat-soluble vitamins A, D, E, and K, plus other micronutrients in vegetables.
- Consuming fat stimulates the burning of body fat.
- Without dietary fat, you'd have to rely on carbs and protein for energy, but if you take in more than a certain amount of carbs, you'll remain on a primarily sugar metabolism, and if you rely on too much protein, you won't feel as well.

Bottom line: there's no other way to get the calories (energy) you need and to switch to a primarily fat metabolism without dietary fat.

FOUR PHASES, FOUR OBJECTIVES

An all-too-common misconception is that the first phase of Atkins, known as Induction, is the whole program. That's undoubtedly where many people get the idea that on Atkins you eat only a small amount of carbs and omit major food groups from your diet. Well, nothing could be further from the truth. Just as you don't go directly from pre-school to third grade, or from seventh grade to high school, each of the four phases has a distinct purpose. And just as with your education, each progressively less restrictive phase builds upon the prior one as it stakes out new territory.

Okay, listen up. Essential to success on Atkins is the process of finding the maximum number of grams of carbs you can consume while continuing to lose weight, keep your appetite under control, and stay alert and energized. This number represents your personal carb balance, which is different for each individual. It also typically increases as you lose weight. To find it, you'll gradually increase both the amount and variety of carbohydrate foods you eat. Learning how to balance your carb intake with continued weight loss is what makes Atkins unique. Then, once you've reached your goal weight, you'll find the maximum number of grams of carbs you can consume while maintaining that weight, staying on top of cravings, and feeling good. This number represents your personal carb tolerance.

In Part II, I'll explain in detail how to do each phase and offer ways to simplify the program. There you'll also learn how to segue naturally from one phase to the next and finally to embark on your new permanent way of eating. But for now let's take a quick snapshot of each of the four phases of the New Atkins Diet.

- **Phase 1: Induction (Kick-Start)**
  How long: A minimum of two weeks, but you may safely follow it for much longer if you have a lot of excess weight to lose

or prefer to lose most of your excess pounds relatively quickly, using the Fast Track (page 101). In this case, you'll stay in this phase until you're 15 pounds from goal weight.

Purpose: Shift your body from burning primarily carbs to burning primarily fat, kick-starting weight loss.

Strategy: Significantly drop your daily Net Carb intake to an average of 20 (no less than 18 and no more than 22) grams of Net Carbs, the level at which almost anyone begins to burn primarily fat.

- **Phase 2: Ongoing Weight Loss (Balancing)**

How long: Typically until you're within 10 pounds of your goal weight, although you can transition to Phase 3 sooner if you're willing to slow the pace of weight loss.

Purpose: Lose most of your excess pounds and find your personal carb balance.

Strategy: Starting at 25 grams of Net Carbs daily, begin to increase overall carb intake in 5-gram increments. This means gradually reintroducing a broader array of carb foods as you step up the Carb Ladder, finding your personal carb balance. It could level off anywhere between 30 and 80 daily grams of Net Carbs or even higher. Your personal number is impacted by your age, gender, activity level, hormonal status, and other factors as you continue to lose weight.

- **Phase 3: Pre-Maintenance (Fine-Tuning)**

How long: Until you've reached your goal weight and maintained it for a month.

Purpose: Trim your final excess pounds, continuing to explore your personal carb balance. Then find your tolerance for carb intake while maintaining your new weight. This phase is a dress rehearsal for Lifetime Maintenance.

Strategy: Gradually increase your daily Net Carb intake in 10-gram (or 5-gram, if you prefer) increments, continuing to reintroduce new carb foods, as long as you continue to slowly lose weight and then to maintain that loss.

- **Phase 4: Lifetime Maintenance**
  How long: Ongoing.
  Purpose: Transition to a permanent way of eating that allows you to maintain your new weight.
  Strategy: Remain in control of your weight by adjusting your carb intake if your carb tolerance changes or you regain a few pounds.

WHAT ARE NET CARBS?

You'll use a carb counter to track your daily carbohydrate intake. The downloadable Atkins Carb Counter is available in a printed version and online, as well as a phone app. You'll be counting grams of Net Carbs, rather than total carbs. How come? Although fiber is a form of carbohydrate, it has no impact on blood sugar levels, so grams of fiber can be subtracted from the total grams of carbs in a serving, leaving only those that impact blood sugar. In the case of low-carb products, sugar alcohols likewise have minimal impact on blood sugar, so they too get a free ride. Here's how it works. Say the total grams of carbs listed on a bar's Nutrition Facts panel is 20, but it contains 10 grams of fiber and 7 grams of sugar alcohols. The Net Carb count would be 3 grams.

THE CARB LADDER

The Carb Ladder (see page 16) offers a logical progression in which to reintroduce carbohydrate foods as you shed pounds. It also makes it easy to segue through the first three phases of the New Atkins Diet and then transition to a lifestyle that allows you to maintain your new weight. Even once you've added back certain foods, you'll eat those on the lower rungs most frequently and those on the higher rungs less often. If you have a low carb tolerance, you may not be able to eat some of the foods on the top rungs, or you can have them only rarely. Atkins products are not listed below because they vary in carb impact; most are acceptable in Phase 1, but check the phase coding on the package to be sure.

STEP UP TO WEIGHT LOSS

The illustration entitled Carb Balancing—Steps to Weight Loss, which appears on page 17, shows how the rungs of the Carb Ladder fit within the three weight-loss phases. Important points to understand:

- On the far right, the daily range of Net Carb intake in grams ranges from 20–70, as indicated by the vertical arrow, corresponding to the rungs of the Carb Ladder.
- The ease with which each individual loses weight varies significantly, so the weight-loss numbers merely illustrate that as pounds melt away, you'll gradually reintroduce categories of carb foods in a certain order.
- The amount of weight you plan to lose may be more or less than the example shown.
- Likewise, the number of daily grams of Net Carbs you'll reach in Phases 2 and 3 may be greater or smaller.
- The horizontal arrows illustrate when to introduce food groups for both the Fast Track and the Slow and Steady path to weight loss.

Phase 1

 Rung 1: Foundation vegetables—leafy greens and other low-carb vegetables

Rung 2: Dairy foods high in fat and low in carbs—cream, sour cream, and most cheeses

Phase 2

 Rung 3: Nuts and seeds* (but not chestnuts)

 Rung 4: Berries, cherries, and melon (but not watermelon)

 Rung 5: Whole-milk yogurt and fresh cheeses such as cottage cheese and ricotta

 Rung 6: Legumes, including chickpeas, lentils, and the like

 Rung 7: Tomato and vegetable juice "cocktail" (plus more lemon and lime juice)

Phases 3 and 4

 Rung 8: Other fruits (but not fruit juices or dried fruits)

Rung 9: Higher-carb vegetables such as winter squash, carrots, and peas

Rung 10: Whole grains

---

* You can add nuts and seeds if you stay in Phase 1 beyond two weeks.

For more detail, see the list of acceptable Phase 1 foods on page 35, acceptable Phase 2 foods on page 110, and acceptable foods for Phases 3 and 4 on page 153. Phase 3 foods are also acceptable in Phase 4.

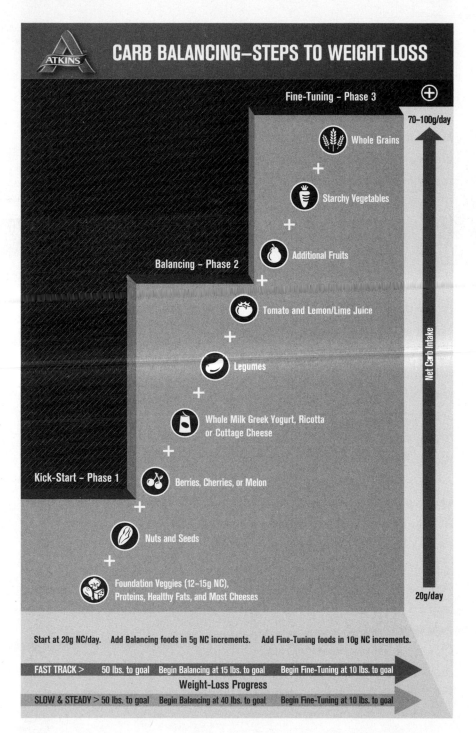

CARB BALANCING—STEPS TO WEIGHT LOSS

Fine-Tuning – Phase 3

70–100g/day

Whole Grains
+
Starchy Vegetables
+
Additional Fruits
+

Balancing – Phase 2

Tomato and Lemon/Lime Juice
+
Legumes
+
Whole Milk Greek Yogurt, Ricotta or Cottage Cheese
+

Kick-Start – Phase 1

Berries, Cherries, or Melon
+
Nuts and Seeds
+
Foundation Veggies (12–15g NC), Proteins, Healthy Fats, and Most Cheeses

Net Carb Intake

20g/day

Start at 20g NC/day.   Add Balancing foods in 5g NC increments.   Add Fine-Tuning foods in 10g NC increments.

FAST TRACK >   50 lbs. to goal   Begin Balancing at 15 lbs. to goal   Begin Fine-Tuning at 10 lbs. to goal

Weight-Loss Progress

SLOW & STEADY > 50 lbs. to goal   Begin Balancing at 40 lbs. to goal   Begin Fine-Tuning at 10 lbs. to goal

FREQUENTLY ASKED QUESTIONS

Q. Can vegetarians do Atkins?
A. Absolutely. It's best to start in Phase 2 so that you can have nuts, fresh cheeses, and legumes as protein sources from the start. See "Atkins for Vegetarians," in Chapter 5. By beginning with 25–30 daily grams of Net Carbs, you'll be able to get sufficient protein. For more specifics, see *The New Atkins for a New You*.

Q. Do I have to eat red meat to do Atkins?
A. No. If you prefer, you can get your protein from poultry and fish.

Q. Can I do Atkins if I'm pregnant?
A. With your doctor's approval, you can follow Phase 4, Lifetime Maintenance. Consume the level of carbs that doesn't stress your blood sugar level but allows for the proper weight gain necessary for a healthy pregnancy. Be sure to consume at least 1,800 calories and at least 50 to 60 grams of Net Carbs daily. Also eat the recommended amount of protein, dairy, and fat along with the recommended minimum of foundation vegetables and two servings of fruit a day, plus a serving of whole grains if your metabolism allows.

Q. Won't eating lots of fat raise my cholesterol level?
A. No. Research shows that people who comply with Phase 1 of the Atkins Diet consistently improve their cholesterol profile, especially their triglycerides. It also raises HDL, the "good" cholesterol. In the context of a low-carb eating program, the fat consumed on Atkins is burned for energy and does not raise the risk for heart disease.

Q. Do I need to count calories on Atkins?
A. Even if you control your carb intake, consuming far too many calories can interfere with weight loss. It's also possible to consume too *few*, which will slow down your metabolism, putting a brake on weight

loss. That said, you're able to eat more (and more-satisfying) food on Atkins than on other weight-loss programs. The minimum daily calorie range for women is 1,500 to 1,800 calories a day and 1,800 to 2,200 for men. There's no need to count calories on Atkins, but if weight loss stalls, do a calorie reality check for few days.

Q. Is there a connection between stress and weight loss? How about sleep?
A. Either can interfere with weight loss. High levels of the stress hormone cortisol stimulate the release of the fat-storing hormone insulin. Yoga, stretching, other low-intensity exercise, and meditation can help minimize stress. Likewise, failing to get at least six hours of sleep a night increases your level of the hunger hormone ghrelin and decreases the level of the hormone leptin, which makes you feel full. People who sleep more tend to be slimmer than people who sleep less.

Q. Is exercise mandatory?
A. No. Exercise isn't essential to lose weight on Atkins. It is, however, effective to help maintain a healthy weight and to potentially break a stall. Combining regular activity with dietary changes has many health benefits and helps elevate mood. Unless you're already engaged in a regular fitness program, it's advisable to wait until you're feeling comfortable with your new eating habits before embarking on a new exercise regimen. If you've already achieved a certain fitness level, feel free to continue your exercise routine.

Q. Can my overweight child do Atkins?
A. It's important to understand that even a heavy youngster is still growing. No one under the age of twelve should be put on any weight-loss diet before consulting with a pediatrician. Meanwhile, weaning your kid off sugar is the single most important thing you can do. If your family starts eating a whole-foods diet, your child will probably lose weight.

In the next chapter, you'll learn how to ready your kitchen before you embark on Atkins, and take care of some other details so you can hit the ground running. And yes, it's time to take that dreaded "before" photo. Believe me, you'll be glad you did a few months from now, when you greet that slim new you in the mirror every morning! But first meet Tori B., who lost an even 100 pounds on Atkins, giving her the courage to initiate many other changes in her life.

A SLIM AND HEALTHY ROLE MODEL
FOR HER DAUGHTERS

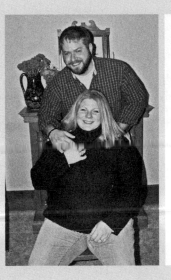

VITAL STATS

Daily Net Carb intake: 20–40
  grams

Age: 37

Height: 5'6"

Before weight: 237 pounds

After weight: 137 pounds

Lost: 100 pounds

Tori B. was the grand prize winner of the 2012 Atkins weight-loss competition. It was a big deal for her to fly from her home in South Barre, Vermont, to Los Angeles with her husband on their prize vacation, where she met with Atkins spokesperson Sharon Osbourne. "I used to be scared of everything before I lost weight, including flying. I'd even worry that I couldn't fit in a roller coaster seat," she recalls. But after losing 100 pounds on Atkins, Tori welcomes challenges and savors every day of her new life, as she explains.

I was never a heavy kid, but after I hit puberty my weight became a problem. You name it, I tried it, but I would always regain the lost pounds. After the birth of Grace, who is now nine years old, I had a miscarriage. I wanted to do everything I could to ensure a healthy infant the next time. Around this time my husband got a new job, and I was in a position to stop working and devote myself to motherhood and getting slim and healthy.

Why did I choose Atkins? I sat down and thought about what I was eating and wrote it all down. It was all carbs, so obviously that was my issue. Also, I wasn't very active before I started Atkins. I was on a high the first day and had already lost 2 pounds by the second day. Two weeks after I started Atkins my energy returned and I felt better emotionally. I started walking three miles every day through Vermont's beautiful countryside. I lost weight consistently, which motivated me to continue. Within three months I'd lost 50 pounds. My husband was very supportive, which also helped. He lost weight without even trying just by eating what I was eating!

At this point I realized I was pregnant again, so I switched to a modified version of Induction with my doctor's approval. Grace now has a five-year-old sister, Anne. After her birth I wanted to achieve a total loss of 100 pounds so I could be a healthy role model for the girls. Of course, I also wanted this for myself. I knew I needed to take care of me so that I'd be there for them for a good long time. With the well-balanced array of foods you eat on Atkins and exercise, those last pounds melted away. There aren't enough words to describe how incredible I feel. Atkins empowered me to live life more fully and try new things, like Zumba. I've have never been so healthy and so in shape. And it's not just me. The whole family skis, snowshoes, and bicycles together.

I hold myself accountable for everything I eat. I weigh myself every day. I figure if I'm going to do it, I'm going to do it right. I never feel hungry as long as I stay away from starches. Mornings are crazy with two kids to get out the door, so I have an Atkins Day Break Chocolate Hazelnut Bar. I call it my "get-up-and-go bar." Then around nine-thirty or ten o'clock I'll have a real breakfast.

My children don't know the unhealthy Mom and don't recognize the old me in pictures. More than ever I feel that little girls need healthy guidance about body image and to be shown by example. And though I started out just wanting to be a role model for our daughters, now my transformation has also influenced my extended family. There's a history of heart disease, high cholesterol, and hypertension, so they were worried about my eating red meat, eggs, and cheese. Now they see that I also eat lots of vegetables and that foods like doughnuts, cookies, and sugary cereals never make it into my house.

Winning the contest was amazing, as was meeting Sharon Osbourne. The old Tori never could have put her story out there by entering the Atkins competition. The Atkins lifestyle is truly a blessing. If you can find it within yourself to take the journey and follow it through, you'll see how fantastic this lifestyle is. If you eat the right foods and exercise, this way of being will change your outlook on life. I couldn't be prouder of where I am today compared to where I started.

MAKE IT EASY

I literally write down everything I eat, even a little piece of Cheddar cheese, in a notebook. That way if I gain a pound or two it's easy to see what caused it. —*T.B.*

CHAPTER 2

PREPARE TO SUCCEED

Now that you know that Atkins is an easy and great-tasting way to lose weight, as well as the basics of how it works, let's get going! Once you finish this chapter, you'll be able to start the New Atkins Diet and begin the exciting process of changing your metabolism, taking control of your appetite, improving your appearance, and boosting your self-image! Let's deal with a few practical matters first, so that you get off on the right foot from the start.

Clearly, having the right food in the fridge, freezer, and pantry is essential, so this chapter includes a list of the kinds of foods you can eat in Phase 1. You'll be amazed and delighted at how many tasty and satisfying choices there are. I'll also introduce you to some exciting new digital tools that will make it easier than ever to slim down on Atkins, and remind you about some of the time-honored aids to help you set your goal weight, track your progress, and achieve your goal.

DOCUMENT THE "BEFORE" YOU

Everyone loves to look at before and after photos, particularly when they reveal an almost unbelievable transformation. You're probably already envisioning the sleeker, sexier, and more energized new you. Hold that image—it's key to making your dream a reality. But let's deal with the current you first. Ask a friend to capture a full-length shot of you, or set it up yourself by using the delayed shutter action feature on your camera. Paste the photo into your journal (or append it to your online journal or save it on your phone; we'll get to that in a moment), noting the date. Or place it where you'll see it several times a day, such as on the refrigerator door or medicine cabinet mirror.

Why is this photo so important? Initially it serves as an ongoing reminder of what you want to change about yourself. As time goes by, it becomes proof positive of your progress. And when you find yourself tempted by a high-carb treat, that "before" photo can help you resolve not to let a moment on your lips become a lifetime on your hips. Believe me, the day will come when you'll find it hard to believe that you were the person in that photo—and what a kick that will be!

WEIGH IN AND MEASURE UP

Just as a "before" photo serves as a baseline, weighing yourself before you begin Atkins allows you to track your progress. Although this is hardly your favorite activity at the moment, I promise you that as the weeks go by, you'll find it an increasingly pleasurable one. You can be nude, in your underwear, or clothed, but do take off your shoes. Ideally, weigh in after you've emptied your bladder and before breakfast. Also measure your chest, waist, hips, and thighs. Enter those baseline numbers in your journal to gauge your progress going forward.

Thereafter, weigh yourself once a week at the same time, using the same scale, if possible, and measure yourself. Why just once a week? It's natural for your weight to fluctuate from day to day and even within a day, depending on your body's natural processes. A weekly weigh-in is a better indicator of how much weight you've lost. Also, checking daily could discourage you when progress is slow or you appear to have regained a pound or two. It's perfectly natural not to lose weight every day no matter how diligently you follow the Atkins program. You may lose nothing for four days, then appear to suddenly lose 2 pounds. Weighing weekly minimizes such natural variations. If you feel compelled to get on the scale every day, weight averaging is another option (see page 46).

SET YOUR GOAL WEIGHT

Don't obsess about a particular number if you don't already have one in mind. Just set a reasonable and realistic goal to aim for. You can always adjust your goal weight as you move through the program. The real objective is to make your goal tangible so that you can visualize the new you waiting to emerge. Once you come up with a number you're comfortable with, enter it in your journal.

If you have a significant amount of weight to lose, you may choose to establish some incremental goals and peg them to specific dates. You'll still keep your ultimate goal front of mind, of course, but every time you shed another 10 or 15 pounds, you'll have reason to celebrate rather than feel overwhelmed by the longer road ahead. This is exactly what Natalie (page 191) did. Her objective of losing 260 pounds was so daunting that she set incremental goals. "That way, every time I lost 5 pounds," she says, "I felt good about myself, and that kept me going."

TO GET RESULTS, GET SPECIFIC

The more quantifiable a goal, the more likely you are to achieve it. No matter how optimistic you are, "I just want to slim down fast" or "I want to lose oodles of pounds" won't fly. Naming your goal weight and adding other specific details, such as why you want to achieve that weight and the time frame in which to do so, makes the goal more tangible and reminds you of why you're going to stay the course. For example:

- "I want to get to 140 pounds so that I can feel comfortable in a bathing suit by the time the pool opens."
- "My goal is to lose 20 pounds by our wedding anniversary so that I can wear that fabulous dress I got on our honeymoon."
- "My daughter is getting married a year from now, and I'm going to be 70 pounds slimmer so I can fit into my old tux when I give her away at the altar."

Come up with your own reasons and enter them in your journal.

STAY REAL

When setting your goal weight, make it achievable. Don't set yourself up for disappointment, or worse, by being overly ambitious. Say you've gained 50 pounds and had two children since you graduated from high school twenty-five years ago. You've just agreed to go to your reunion in three months' time. It's unlikely that you can meet a goal of losing that 50 pounds in that time frame. Even with a realistic timeline, understand that you may not be able to achieve the same weight at age forty-three that you were at eighteen. Your metabolism is almost certain to change over the years. A better approach would be to set a more reasonable goal, such as 10 pounds heavier than your high school graduation weight. When you reach that weight, celebrate your success, and consider resetting your goal.

ASSEMBLE YOUR ATKINS TOOL KIT

You need just four items to track your weight, measurements, and carb intake, Having these on hand from the start will allow you to track and record your progress.

1. *A scale.* No need for any fancy bells and whistles. If necessary, weigh in at your office, health club, or a pharmacy.

2. *A cloth measuring tape.* Inches are as important as pounds in tracking your progress and may show changes before weight loss registers.

3. *Atkins Carb Counter and Acceptable Foods List.* Download this handy, pocket-size list (referred to as the Atkins Carb Counter from here on) of acceptable foods for each phase of Atkins, along with the Net Carb counts for hundreds of whole foods, Atkins products, and meals and beverages at popular restaurant chains. You'll find it at atkins.com. This information is also available for your smartphone.

4. *A journal or notebook.* You'll be entering your weight and measurements weekly, but recording your food intake and Net Carb count daily. Research consistently shows that people who journal lose more weight than those who don't. *The New Atkins for a New You Workbook* is specially designed to comply with the Atkins program, but a simple notebook can do the trick as well. Or use the Atkins online tools. Remember, these numbers are for your eyes only. Pretty soon you'll see the weight and measurements numbers going down, down, down. Also, feel free to record your thoughts and feelings about your weight-loss journey.

EXPLORE THE ATKINS ONLINE RESOURCES AND MOBILE APP

In addition to the items in your basic tool kit, go to atkins.com to access these resources:

- A carb counter that lists hundreds of foods and tracks your daily carb intake
- Additional meal planners, including a customizable program that incorporates your food preferences

- Online trackers for your weight and measurements, as well as one for exercise
- A BMI calculator
- The Atkins database of more than sixteen hundred recipes, with customized shopping lists for each recipe

If you have a smartphone, download the free Atkins app. These features make it easier than ever to follow the program, especially when you're on the move:

- *Food Search.* Nutritional information on hundreds of items in the supermarket, restaurant meals, more than sixteen hundred Atkins recipes, and Atkins products. Simply enter a keyword or scan in the UPC label.
- *Progress Tracker.* Helps you to monitor your progress by tallying your daily Net Carb intake and weight, and calculating how close you are to your goal weight.
- *Phase Overview.* A listing of the acceptable foods for each of the four Atkins phases.
- *Daily Food Plan.* Both recommended and customizable plans (based on your carb intake and food preferences) for each phase
- *Recipe Database.* Search hundreds of recipes by phase or key ingredients.
- *Dining Out Guide.* Locates places with meals in your carb intake range. Search based on meal type, restaurant name, and location.

BUILD YOUR ATKINS LIBRARY

Want to learn more? If you're interested in delving deeper into why Atkins works and the research that validates this approach, check out *The New Atkins for a New You*. And if cooking is your thing, you'll find two hundred recipes for delectable low-carb meals that you can put together in thirty minutes or less in *The New Atkins for a New You Cookbook*. Both print and electronic versions are available at bookstores everywhere, as well as on Amazon.

MAKE YOUR KITCHEN ATKINS FRIENDLY

Unless you have superior self-control, it's best to remove temptation in the form of high-carb foods, at least for the first few weeks on Atkins. Once you've switched over to burning primarily fat for energy, your desire for chips, crackers, cookies, doughnuts, candy bars, and so forth will be suppressed. Hard to believe, but true! There are also plenty of tasty low-carb substitutes for most of them. But for now, removing problematic foods (or setting them apart from other foods) is the best strategy, perhaps by giving them to a friend, a neighbor, or even a food pantry. That means breakfast cereal, bread, pasta, sweets, and anything else made with refined grains and/or sugar. But out with the old unacceptable foods is only half the strategy, the other half is having the right foods in the house.

SHOP FOR SUCCESS

The last thing you want is to find that there's nothing in the house you can eat on your first day on Atkins. The components of a low-carb meal aren't unusual or exotic. With the very occasional exception, everything you need is available at your supermarket. Specialty items such as starch-free thickener for making low-carb gravy can be easily ordered online. To make things super easy for you, we've come up with meal plans for your first two weeks on Atkins (see pages 62–65 and 88–91), along with shopping lists (pages 66 and 92), so that you'll have everything you need to hit the ground running. No later than the day before you start Atkins, photocopy the first shopping list and get yourself to the store.

WHAT TO LOOK FOR ON A FOOD LABEL

Being able to understand the data on a food label will help you steer clear of high-carb or otherwise problematic ingredients. Food manufacturers don't make it easy for you, so listen up. There are two parts to a label, both of which contain vital information:

- *The Nutrition Facts panel* lists the serving size, number of calories in a serving—a 12-ounce bottle of soda or another beverage may actually be two or more servings—and the amounts of macronutrients, including carbs, fat, and protein, both in grams and as a percentage of the recommended Daily Value. Ditto for certain micronutrients, including fiber and some vitamins. Remember to subtract grams of fiber (and sugar alcohols, in the case of low-carb foods) from total grams of carbs to get the Net Carbs. Our example, for a major brand of creamy peanut butter, lists 0 trans fats per serving and 3 grams of sugar.

- *The ingredient list* includes everything in the product, in order of volume. Here's where you might find one of the umpteen aliases for sugar (see page 70)—in this case, both sugar and molasses appear—or other unacceptable ingredients. Although the Nutrition Facts panel lists 0 grams of trans fats per serving—a loophole allows this as long as there is less than 0.5 grams per serving—the ingredient list includes another unacceptable ingredient, hydrogenated vegetable oil, aka trans fats.

Nutrition Facts	
Serving Size 2 Tbsp (32g)	
Amount per Serving	
Calories 190	
Calories from Fat 130	
	% Daily Value*
Total Fat 16g	24%
Saturated Fat 2.5g	13%
Trans Fat 0g	
Cholesterol 0mg	0%
Sodium 140mg	6%
Total Carbohydrate 8g	3%
Dietary Fiber 2g	9%
Sugars 3g	
Protein 7g	
Vitamin E 10%	Iron 4%
Niacin 20%	Riboflavin 2%

Not a significant source of vitamin A, vitamin C and calcium.

*Percent Daily Values are based on a 2,000 calorie diet.

Ingredients:
MADE FROM ROASTED PEANUTS AND SUGAR, CONTAINS 2% OR LESS OF: MOLASSES, FULLY HYDROGENATED VEGETABLE OILS (RAPESEED AND SOYBEAN), MONO AND DIGLYCERIDES, SALT.

Kosher Information:
Ⓤ

HOW TO ID ADDED SUGAR

Packaged food labels don't make it easy for you to judge whether the sugar in a product is added or naturally occurring. You can distinguish whether a product has naturally occurring sugar, added sugar, or both. But when it contains both kinds, there's no way to know how much of each, as this example shows.

1. The Nutrition Facts panel lists the number of grams of sugar in a serving. In the case of a 6-ounce container of Dannon Fruit on the Bottom Mixed Berry Yogurt, which is made with low-fat milk, the label lists 27 grams of sugar.

2. When you look at the list of ingredients, you'll see that the first ingredient is low-fat milk, which contains naturally occurring sugars. But, tellingly, fructose syrup and sugar are listed before blueberries, which is followed by high-fructose corn syrup. Ingredients are listed in order of highest content, meaning there are more of these two added sugars than a key fruit.

3. So we've learned that there are lots of added sugars in this supposedly nutritious food, but we have no way to quantify the added sugar as opposed to the naturally occurring sugar.

This single example makes a strong case for having the Nutrition Facts panel distinguish between the two kinds of sugar.

THE SCOOP ON SUGAR: A GLOSSARY OF SWEETS

The terminology used to describe the absence or presence of sugar can be confusing, especially when you're new to low-carb eating and trying to make smart buying decisions. A few definitions should cut through the doublespeak.

- *Added sugar* is not integral to the product. An apple comes by sugar naturally in the form of fructose, but when that fructose is used in a cookie, for example, it constitutes added sugar. You want to avoid *all* added sugars, sometimes referred to as "hidden sugars."

- *Low (or reduced) sugar* suggests that there is less added sugar than is typical in a product, but it still contains added sugar. Avoid such products.

- *Natural sugar* is a term likely to appear on the labels of health food store products. Whether honey, molasses, or agave syrup, natural sugar is still sugar.

- *No added sugar* means that a food contains only integral sugars. Examples would be any raw or cooked vegetable, fruit, whole grains, or unflavored dairy products.

- *No table sugar* merely means that a food contains no sucrose, but very likely it contains other natural or processed sugars. Again, sugar is sugar.

- *Sugar free* asserts that a food contains no natural sugars, whether integral or added. Only oils, fats, and a few types of meat and other protein sources are naturally sugar free.

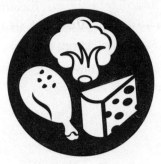

ACCEPTABLE PHASE 1 FOODS

Now let's preview the delectable foods you get to eat in Phase 1 (Kick-Start), along with a few to avoid. Rather than overwhelm you with the hundreds of vegetables and dozens of cheeses, for example, I've listed just a few common ones here. For more extensive lists, and for serving sizes complete with grams of Net Carbs, download the Atkins Carb Counter, which includes Acceptable Food Lists at atkins.com or use the mobile app.

PROTEIN FOODS

- All fish, whether fresh, frozen, canned, or vacuum packed . . . except:
  - Anything deep-fried, stuffed, breaded, battered, or coated in flour
  - Pickled or creamed herring that contains added sugar
- Shellfish, including crab, oysters, shrimp, and clams . . . except:
  - Anything deep-fried, breaded, battered, or coated in flour
  - And limit oysters and mussels, which contain carbs
- All poultry . . . except:
  - Chicken nuggets, breaded cutlets, or anything that has been deep-fried, stuffed, breaded, battered, or coated in flour
  - Chicken or turkey sausages that contain fillers or other high-carb ingredients

- Beef, lamb, pork, and all other meats, including game . . . except:
  - Products that contain fillers and/or added sugar, including hot dogs,* sausage,* salami,* and bologna*
  - Meatballs, meatloaf, Salisbury steak, and anything stuffed with bread crumbs
- Eggs prepared in any fashion (each egg contains 0.6 gram of Net Carbs)

OILS AND FATS

No need to count carbs here. Oils are one of the few foods that contain just a single macronutrient: fat! A typical serving size is 1 tablespoon. Choose from among:

- Butter, stick or whipped
- Canola oil
- Coconut oil
- Flaxseed oil
- Grapeseed oil
- Mayonnaise†
- Olive oil
- High-oleic safflower oil
- Sesame oil

CHEESE

Most cheeses contain less than 1 gram of Net Carbs per ounce and are fine in this phase, with the exception of cottage cheese and ricotta, which you'll be able to add in Phase 2. Don't exceed 4 ounces a day, the

---

* We recommend nitrate-free products whenever possible.
† Mayonnaise contains a minute amount of carbs. Choose a brand made with canola or high-oleic safflower oil, not soybean or vegetable oil, whenever possible.

equivalent of four individually wrapped slices or cubes the size of large dice. A tablespoon or two of any grated cheese contains a negligible amount of carbs. Select whole-milk products. Avoid low-fat cheeses, "diet" cheese, "cheese products" such as Velveeta and Cheez Whiz, and whey cheese and any cheese flavored with fruit. Common cheeses are listed below. Consult the Atkins Carb Counter for a more extensive list.

- Blue cheese
- Brie
- Cheddar or Colby
- Cream cheese, full-fat or plain
- Feta
- Goat (chèvre)
- Gouda
- Havarti
- Jarlsberg
- Laughing Cow
- Mozzarella, whole-milk
- Parmesan
- Romano
- String

ADDITIONAL DAIRY PRODUCTS AND DAIRY SUBSTITUTES

Feel free to use up to 1½ ounces daily or a total of 2–3 tablespoons sour cream, unsweetened whipped cream, and liquid cream or half-and-half in your coffee or tea. Most so-called creamers are full of sugar or high-fructose corn syrup, and all too often they contain unhealthy trans fats as well. However, we've found a few unsweetened nondairy "creamers" without these problematic ingredients. A tablespoon of each contains no more than 1 gram of Net Carbs. See the Atkins Carb Counter for more details.

- Heavy cream, liquid or whipped
- Light cream
- Half-and-half
- Sour cream, full-fat
- Unsweetened or Sugar-Free MimicCreme Almond & Cashew Creme
- Unsweetened Original So Delicious Coconut Milk "Creamer"

Milk is off the menu for the time being, but you can have a cup of several different milk substitutes at 1–2 grams of Net Carbs. All should be plain (unflavored) and sugar free:

- Almond milk
- Coconut milk beverage (not canned coconut milk)
- Soy milk

FOUNDATION VEGETABLES

There is a wealth of veggies acceptable in Phase 1, but we'll keep the list to a minimum for simplicity's sake. They include salad greens and other salad fixings, as well as vegetables that are typically cooked. Your daily minimum of 12–15 grams of Net Carbs translates to about 6 cups leafy greens and 2 cups cooked veggies. (If you're not sure how to get all those veggies in, see the meal plans in the following chapters.) Try to have both types each day, but have more salad veggies and cut back on cooked ones if you prefer. Frozen veggies are fine.

SALAD VEGETABLES A cup of each of the following raw salad greens comes in at less than 1 gram of Net Carbs:

- Arugula
- Cabbage

- Endive
- Lettuce, all types
- Spinach
- Sprouts, all kinds
- Watercress

OTHER SALAD VEGETABLES These are usually slightly higher in carbs. Consult the Atkins Carb Counter for more details on serving sizes and carb counts.

- Hass avocados (the dark green or black ones)
- Bamboo shoots, canned
- Bell peppers, any color
- Celery
- Cucumber
- Mushrooms
- Olives, black or green
- Onions
- Pickles, dill or sour
- Radishes, daikon
- Scallions
- Tomatoes

VEGETABLES TYPICALLY COOKED Half a cup of the following cooked veggies contain no more than 3 grams of Net Carbs. (Be sure to measure them after cooking rather than before.) Those with an asterisk have considerably less.

- Asparagus
- Broccoli
- Cauliflower*
- Chard*
- Eggplant

- Green beans
- Kale
- Mushrooms
- Okra
- Sauerkraut*
- Spaghetti squash
- Spinach*
- Zucchini and other summer squash*
- Turnips

BEVERAGES

Water can be bottled, filtered, mineral, spring, sparkling, or from the tap. Jazz up H2O with a couple of tablespoons of lemon and/or lime juice, if you wish. Most vitamin waters are full of added sugar (see "The Scoop on Sugar: Multiple Aliases" on page 70), but a few brands with acceptable sweeteners have zero grams of carbs. Ditto for canned or bottled iced teas, but always check the Nutrition Facts panel to uncover any added sugar. You can also have hot cocoa mixes sweetened with noncaloric sweeteners and mixed with water (and a splash of cream) instead of milk.

- Coffee (caffeinated or decaf, hot or iced) and espresso
- Tea (caffeinated or decaf); sugar-free iced tea (brewed, bottled, or canned)
- Herb teas without added sugar
- Club soda and seltzer (plain and flavored)
- Diet cola, ginger ale, root beer, birch beer, and other sodas
- Sugar-free fruit refreshers
- Sugar-free tonic
- Sugar-free beverage mixes such as Kool-Aid, Crystal Light, and True Lemon

CONDIMENTS AND SEASONINGS

Such flavor enhancers give zest to meals. All fresh herbs are acceptable in this phase and contain virtually no carbs. So are small amounts of dried herbs, including basil, bay leaves, chives, coriander, cumin, oregano, rosemary, thyme, and others, plus salt and pepper. Most spices and spice mixes such as chili powder, curry powder, and crab/shrimp boil mix are fine, but avoid spice mixes that contain added sugar. Again, this list gives just a small taste of the condiments and seasonings you can use in Induction.

- Bacon pieces
- Celery salt
- Chile peppers
- Garlic
- Ginger root
- Italian seasoning
- Lemon or orange peel, grated
- Paprika
- Red pepper flakes
- Liquid Smoke
- Mrs. Dash
- Mustard (without added sugar)
- Poultry seasoning
- Spike

SAUCES

This category is a bit of a minefield. While one brand of, say, barbecue sauce may be made without sugar, another may be swimming in it. Check the Nutrition Facts panel carefully for added sugars as well as flour and other starches. In cases where the range of carbs can be significant, we've listed acceptable brands (which are often specialty products sweetened with sucralose, stevia, or xylitol). A tablespoon of any of these sauces should not contain more than 1 gram of Net Carbs.

- Alfredo sauce
- Barbecue sauce (Hallman's or Walden Farms)
- Buffalo chicken wing sauce (Beano's)
- Cocktail/seafood sauce (Walden Farms)
- Enchilada sauce (Las Palmas)
- Fish sauce
- Garlic sauce
- Horseradish sauce
- Hot sauce (Tabasco)
- Salsa
- Taco sauce, green or red
- Ketchup (Walden Farms)
- Pesto sauce
- Pasta or pizza sauce (Rao's Sensitive Formula Marinara Sauce, Walden Farms)
- Sofrito
- Soy sauce or tamari (San-J tamari, Seal Sama sugar-free)
- Steak sauce and marinade (Trinity Hill)

Tomato sauce, canned or stewed tomatoes, tomato puree, and tomato paste are all acceptable in Induction, as long as they contain no added sugar. Muir Glen is one such brand.

SALAD DRESSINGS

Any prepared salad dressing without added sugar and no more than 3 grams of Net Carbs per 2-tablespoon serving is acceptable. A lower-carb option is to make your own vinaigrette with olive oil plus either vinegar, lemon juice, or lime juice.

- Blue cheese
- Caesar
- Italian
- Ranch
- Vinaigrette

You can also have up to 2 tablespoons lemon or lime juice a day.

NONCALORIC SWEETENERS

Count each packet as 1 gram of Net Carbs, and consume no more than three per day. Although the sweeteners themselves contain no carbs, the powdered agent that keeps them from clumping has a small amount.

- Splenda (sucralose)
- Truvia or SweetLeaf (natural products made from stevia)
- Sweet'n Low (saccharin)
- Xylitol (available in health food stores and some supermarkets)

ATKINS LOW-CARB PRODUCTS

All Atkins products are coded for appropriate phases. Bars and shakes acceptable for this phase contain no more than 3 grams of Net Carbs. Because they are meal substitutes, the Atkins frozen meals, which contain from 4–7 grams of Net Carbs, are all acceptable for Induction. (Some of the frozen meals contain less than 3 grams of Net Carbs from a small amount of Atkins Cuisine Penne Pasta.) In this phase, you can also have:

- Atkins Advantage Snack Bars with 2 or 3 grams of Net Carbs
- All Atkins Advantage Meal Bars
- All Atkins Advantage Ready-to-Drink Shakes

- Atkins Day Break Bars with 2 or 3 grams of Net Carbs
- All Atkins Endulge Bars (if your carb allotment allows)

You can also eat certain other low-carb foods so long as they contain no more than 3 grams of Net Carbs per serving.

GROCERY STORE TIPS

What if cooking from scratch is not your thing or you rarely have the time? Not to worry. This book is all about making Atkins easy. In addition to the delectable Atkins meals, some of which are suitable for breakfast and others for lunch or dinner, and other products, consider these options:

- Mine the frozen-foods section for products such as burgers in single servings, chicken tenders, and lots of different veggies. Some come in their own steaming bags that you can puncture and pop in the microwave oven. No pots to wash!
- Look in the same section for fish fillets (the unbreaded kind), scallops, and shrimp in parchment packets for super-quick meals.
- Visit the deli section for precooked roasted or grilled chicken and turkey that comes in chunks or slices. They're great for tossing together a stir-fry, a main-dish salad, or another no-cook or easy-cook meal in no time.
- You can even find cooked hard-boiled eggs in the dairy department of the supermarket.

We'll explore these options in greater detail, along with lots more ideas, in Chapter 9.

THE BEST TIME TO START ATKINS

No matter how eager you are to start paring pounds, starting today or tomorrow might not be the best idea. Why wait? If you work outside the home, you might be better off waiting for the weekend, when you have more control of your time and when and what you eat. Or spend the weekend getting ready and turn a new page on Monday morning. You also don't want any added stressors occurring simultaneously. So if it's exam week, crunch time at the office, or the first week of a new job, or if your kid is sick with the flu, hold off. Likewise, if you're leaving on vacation or celebrating the holidays, when temptation is everywhere, you may want to wait until you can focus on your new way of eating.

That said, don't fall into the trap of always finding an excuse to put off starting until tomorrow or next week. There will always be social and work situations to navigate and temptation wherever you turn. Pick a date and stick to it. You'll be proud of your resolve. Get used to that feeling!

DISCUSS MEDICATIONS WITH YOUR DOCTOR

If you're taking certain prescription drugs, check with your physician *before* starting Atkins. Insulin, some antidepressants, steroids, and beta-blockers can interfere with weight loss. He or she may be able to change the dosage or substitute another drug. If you're taking diuretic medications for high blood pressure, losing water weight and then fat may necessitate a reduced dosage. Check your blood pressure regularly and report any change immediately. Finally, your blood sugar level will begin to self-regulate on Atkins, so if you're taking insulin, you'll have to reduce your dosage to avoid your blood sugar dropping too low. Test your blood sugar level regularly and work closely with your physician.

FREQUENTLY ASKED QUESTIONS

Q. How do I incorporate Atkins products into my eating plan?

A. Atkins products can make all the difference in being able to stay with the program regardless of where you are at mealtime or snack time. But convenience foods shouldn't replace foundation vegetables and other whole foods. Make sure to consume at least 12 and preferably 15 of your allotted 20 daily Net Carb grams in the form of foundation vegetables, some of which can be in the frozen meals.

Q. Do I have to take vitamin supplements on Atkins?

A. You'll be eating foods full of vitamins, minerals, and antioxidants, but it's still difficult to ensure you're getting all the nutrients you need on a daily basis, so it is just a good insurance policy to take a few supplements. In addition to a daily multivitamin-mineral supplement (without iron unless you're anemic), I advise taking additional vitamin D and omega-3 fatty acids (unless you're having two or more servings of fatty fish a week). Significant weight loss reduces your stores of omega-3s. Your body makes vitamin D after exposure to sunlight, but levels can diminish in winter or during overcast periods.

Q. What is weight averaging?

A. Your weight naturally fluctuates from day to day, which is why I recommend weighing in once a week. If you must weigh yourself daily, add that number to those from the two previous days, then divide by three to get your average weight. You can even do this on your cell phone. A running three-day average gives you a better sense of your progress than your weight on any single day.

Q. Which sugar substitutes are suitable for beverages and which for cooking?

A. Packets and liquid dispensers are handy for sweetening beverages. The granular forms of sucralose and xylitol sold in a bag or box can be used for cooking.

• • •

Now let's move on to Part II, "It's Easy to Become the New You," where we'll examine each of the four phases of the Atkins Diet, starting with Phase 1, which kick-starts weight loss, so you can see results pronto! But first, take a few minutes to be inspired by Charity W., who lost 135 pounds on Atkins, enduring two extended periods when the scale wouldn't budge. In her determination to reach her goal, Charity would begin each day repeating, "I can do this." And so she did.

THE SECOND TIME'S A CHARM

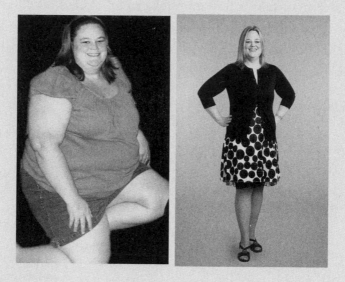

VITAL STATS

Daily Net Carb intake: 20–50
  grams
Age: 37
Height: 5'4"

Before weight: 285 pounds
After weight: 150 pounds
Lost: 135 pounds

Charity W. knew that Atkins works. She'd lost 40 pounds in three months on the program before her 2004 wedding, but after the honeymoon she returned to her old ways, eating lots of pasta and bread, plus "tons of sugar." The Minneapolis, Minnesota, resident also loves to bake. So back came the pounds and with them health issues. Charity takes it from here.

In 2010 I visited my in-laws, when photos of the whole family were taken. When the pictures arrived I was very unhappy with them. Was I really that big? I had heard that Atkins had changed, placing more emphasis on vegetables. I read *The New Atkins for a New You*, and I thought, "I can do that, and I can do it for the rest of my life." The first month was the hardest. I had headaches, but drinking broth helped, and by the second week they were gone. Every day when I woke up I would say, "I can do it!" I even wrote these words on my bathroom mirror so they were just about the first thing I saw each morning. By the end of the month, I'd lost 15 pounds.

After two weeks on Induction, I added nuts. After twelve weeks I stalled at 263 pounds and realized I was overdoing the cheese, so I cut back to an ounce a day. Still the number on the scale wouldn't budge. I was so disheartened that I went to the Atkins Community for help. The advice and encouragement I got were terrific. I stuck with protein, fat, vegetables, and nuts. That did the trick. In one week my body played catch-up, dropping 4 pounds. After six months in Phase 1, I moved to Phase 2, adding berries and yogurt. I found the berries were causing cravings, so I knocked them out.

Within six months I'd lost 55 pounds, and eleven months after starting I hit the big number: 100 pounds gone. Until this point, I hadn't done any exercise. I hit another plateau during the holidays, and started working out. Nonetheless, I stayed at 185 for eight endless weeks. But I stayed with Atkins and the workouts. When I finally hit my goal of 150 pounds after about sixteen months, it was one of my happiest days of my life. I did it! Just like I knew I could.

I still love to bake, but I've made some big changes. Instead of wheat flour, I now use almond and coconut flours, plus flax-seed meal for tortillas. My favorite sweeteners are stevia and sugar alcohols, but I use as little as possible. Spices are very important for low-carb baking. I love to try new recipes and have found some great ones on the Atkins website.

I'm very careful about portions. I'll put one or two cookies in a freezer bag and have only that much for a snack. I've also found my carb tolerance allows me to eat berries and even half an apple, but I stay away from rice, potatoes, and any processed food.

Losing weight has changed a lot of other things in my life. I'd had gestational diabetes in both my pregnancies and been plagued with irritable bowel syndrome and acid reflux for years. Both are now gone. I'm at the gym five or six times a week, often for two or three hours at a time, swimming and doing weight and elliptical training. I used to roller-skate when I was younger, and now I'm doing it again. I also spend more time playing with my kids. Life is good. And Atkins helped me get there.

MAKE IT EASY

Here's my recipe for quick egg muffins. Cut up a precooked sausage link and place it in a greased muffin tin with grated cheese and minced onion and peppers—sauté the onion and peppers first. Whisk an egg and pour it over the other ingredients. Bake at 350°F until set. Make a batch and freeze in individual plastic freezer bags. Defrost the night before or in the microwave. —*C.W.*

PART II

IT'S EASY TO BECOME THE NEW YOU

CHAPTER 3

YOUR FIRST WEEK ON ATKINS

Now that you understand how the program works and the kinds of foods you'll be eating, I have a few questions for you:

- Are you ready to have the body you've always dreamed of?
- Are you ready to eat three yummy meals and two satisfying snacks a day, and still shed pounds?
- Are you ready to actually get your appetite under control once and for all?
- Are you ready to reinvent yourself?

If your answer to all four questions is yes—and of course it is—congratulations on taking this important first step toward turning your dreams into reality! And welcome to your first week on Atkins. The purpose of the first phase of the program, known as Induction, is to kick-start weight loss. Although it takes a few days to actually start losing fat pounds—water pounds come off first—you'll almost certainly see real results by the end of the week. Some people lose as much as a pound a day.

You'll achieve this amazing feat by dropping your carbohydrate intake to a level at which almost anyone starts burning primarily fat
for energy after a few days. Then, like magic, those excess pounds
begin to vanish. Even if you have just a little weight to lose or you've
decided to begin in a later phase of Atkins, understanding how this
first phase works gives you a solid grounding in the whole program.
Doing Atkins right from the beginning will bring faster and more impressive results. My job is to make that as easy as possible for you.

In this chapter you'll find a couple of meal plans for Week 1 (see
pages 62 and 64), one with a companion shopping list (page 66) incor-
porating foods suitable for Phase 1 (the first rung on the Carb Ladder—
see page 16), as well as more advice on what to eat and how to prepare
it. We'll also go into greater detail about why you should be eating
certain foods and passing on others. Finally, we'll discuss some small
changes that can spell the difference between immediate success and
a frustrating delay.

TEN SIMPLE STEPS FOR SUCCESS

Follow these guidelines to get off on the right foot from day one:

1. *Have three meals and two snacks a day.* Never starve yourself
   or go more than three or four waking hours without eating.
   If you prefer, have five or even six small meals. You never
   want to allow yourself to become ravenously hungry. That can
   open the door to eating whatever's at hand. Not a good idea!
2. *Consume 20 grams of Net Carbs a day.* Of these, 12–15 grams
   should be in the form of foundation vegetables (see page 38).
   It's fine to average 20 grams a day over several days, but don't go
   below 18 grams or above 22 on a single day. Dropping below 18
   probably won't make you lose weight any faster and is unlikely
   to satisfy your vegetable requirement. Going above 22 could

interfere with triggering weight loss. Select carb foods from the list of Phase 1 acceptable foods in the previous chapter.

3. *Eat sufficient protein at every meal.* As you now know, protein plays a key role in weight loss and protects lean muscle mass, so you lose only fat.

4. *Don't restrict fats.* Consuming fat is essential to slimming down on Atkins. Fat also heightens the flavor of foods and enables your body to absorb certain vitamins. Always accompany a carb snack with either fat or protein. For example, have cucumber slices with a piece of cheese.

5. *Drink at least eight 8-ounce glasses of water daily.* Two of these can be replaced with coffee or tea. Another 2 cups can be replaced with beef, chicken, or vegetable broth (not the low-sodium kind).

6. *Avoid dehydration or electrolyte imbalance.* The perfectly normal initial loss of water weight can lead to light-headedness and other symptoms and rob you of energy. These symptoms disappear once you're burning primarily fat, but in the meantime, be sure to consume sufficient salt in the form of salty broth, salt, tamari, or soy sauce. For more, see "Stop Certain Symptoms Before They Start" on page 68.

7. *Watch out for hidden carbs.* Read food labels carefully, particularly on condiments. In restaurants, ask for oil and vinegar to dress your salad, request sauces on the side, and feel free to ask the server what's in a dish.

8. *Use sugar substitutes—in moderation.* (See "Noncaloric Sweeteners" on page 43.) That means no more than three packets a day.

9. *Use only Atkins low-carb products.* Most of these have been tested to ensure that their impact on your blood sugar level is minimal. The majority of them are coded for Phase 1.

10. *Eat nothing that isn't on the list of Phase 1 acceptable foods.*

A WEALTH OF CHOICES

From the start, you can eat a wide range of foods, including almost all forms of animal protein, as well as several vegetarian ones. Pick your favorites, select budget-conscious cuts, or have "meatless Mondays," if you wish. Most animal sources contain no carbs, with a few exceptions noted in the Phase 1 acceptable foods list.

Since fat is *not* a no-no on Atkins, you can stir-fry meats, poultry, fish, and vegetables in oil, serve protein dishes with cream sauces, top veggies with a pat of butter, and use oil-based dressings on your salad—all without guilt. However, you don't want to go overboard on protein or fat either, as we'll explain. Most of your initial carbs will come from foundation vegetables, but there are also many condiments and beverages you can enjoy. You'll be counting grams of Net Carbs—remember, that's grams of fiber (and sugar alcohols in the case of some low-carb foods) subtracted from total carb grams.

THE RIGHT FATS . . .

Your objective is to consume a broad variety of natural fats with the most health benefits. So which should you be eating—or not?

- Dress salads and veggies with extra-virgin olive oil; virgin olive oil is fine for cooking.
- Cook with canola and most nut oils. Like olives and avocados, they reduce levels of "bad" (LDL) cholesterol and triglycerides. High-oleic safflower oil handles high heat well.
- You can also cook with butter or coconut oil, and top veggies and other foods with butter.
- Have two to three weekly servings of fish and/or shellfish.
- Snack on olives and avocados, and include them in salads. Nuts and seeds also make great snacks and garnishes once you've been on Atkins for two weeks.

- There's no need to cut the fat off meat or remove the skin from poultry, but you can do so if you prefer.

Avoid:

- Any oil that has been subjected to nutrient-destroying high heat during processing. Instead, look for cold-pressed or expeller-pressed oils and store them away from heat sources and direct light.
- Trans fats, which are vegetable oils that have been blasted with hydrogen gas to make them shelf stable, have been linked to an increased risk of heart disease and other health problems. The words *hydrogenated* or *partially hydrogenated* on the list of ingredients mean that a product contains trans fats. In addition to most shortenings and some margarines, many commercial baked goods contain trans fats.

. . . AND THE RIGHT AMOUNTS

The trick is to consume enough fat to keep your fat-burning engine humming along, but not so much as to create a calorie bomb, which may interfere with weight loss. As with protein, the correct intake depends in part on your gender and size. Small women may need less and big guys may need more, but follow these guidelines and you should be fine. You can replace one with another—another ounce of cream, for example, in lieu of an egg. In addition to the fat in your daily servings of fish, shellfish, poultry, and meat, here's a typical day's fat intake:

- 2 or 3 eggs
- 2 tablespoons olive or another oil for dressing salads and cooking
- 1 tablespoon butter
- 1 ounce cream

- 2 ounces cheese
- 10 olives and/or ½ Hass avocado
- 2 ounces seeds or nuts (after first two weeks on Induction)

There's no need to eat only lean cuts of meat and white-meat poultry. Nor must you remove the skin from chicken or turkey or cut off fat on a steak or pork chop. If you prefer to, fine, but if so, replace the fat with other natural fats.

PORTION CONTROL

Overestimating serving sizes is a common mistake people make on any weight-loss program. Eat too large a serving of any carb food and you'll likely exceed the initial recommended daily 20 grams of Net Carbs. Overly large portions of protein foods can also stall weight loss. If you don't have a food scale or don't want to bother with measuring spoons or cups to track your carb and protein intake, take another approach. Use the familiar visuals listed below to estimate a 4- or 6-ounce portion of meat or fish, or a ½-cup portion of steamed spinach or sautéed zucchini. (Foods marked with an asterisk will be introduced in later phases.)

FOOD	VISUAL
4 ounces meat, poultry, fish tofu, etc.	A smartphone
6 ounces meat, poultry, fish, tofu, etc.	A hockey puck
8 ounces meat, poultry, tofu, etc.	A slim paperback book
1 ounce hard cheese	A large dice
1 cup salad greens	A baseball
½ cup cooked vegetables	A lightbulb or billiard ball
¼ cup cooked legumes*	An egg
2 tablespoons nut butter*	A golf ball
½ cup cooked grains*	A tennis ball

WHY SO MANY VEGETABLES?

If you came to Atkins thinking it was all about beef and bacon, you may be surprised to find yourself eating more veggies than you ever did before. Initially you'll be eating primarily what we call foundation vegetables, those with a lower carb content and often a higher fiber count than starchy vegetables higher up the Carb Ladder. Powerhouses of vitamins, minerals, and disease-combatting antioxidants, vegetables are also full of fiber that helps:

- Fill you up, blunting your appetite for higher-carb foods
- Lower cholesterol
- Prevent constipation and maintain GI health

The water content of vegetables, particularly foundation vegetables, also helps keep you well hydrated and replaces electrolytes dissolved in the fluids being washed from your body as you shed the first water pounds. Steaming is a quick and simple way to cook veggies, especially if you microwave them right in the special plastic bag in which some frozen products are sold. Or steam fresh or frozen veggies in a steamer basket. You can also sauté or grill veggies, but never boil them (unless you're making soup), which destroys nutrients.

MAKE IT EASY

To avoid waste from spoilage if you're not cooking many meals at home, you may be better off purchasing frozen veggies and confining your fresh choices to salad vegetables.

WHICH CARBS ARE OFF-LIMITS FOR NOW?

Now that you know what you can eat in the first few weeks on Atkins, let's look at which foods to avoid:

- Fruit (other than rhubarb, which is really a vegetable). Avocados, olives, and tomatoes—all of which are actually fruit—are fine.
- Fruit juice (other than 2 tablespoons lemon and/or lime juice a day).
- Caloric sodas.
- Bread, pasta, muffins, tortillas, chips, and any other food made with flour or other grain products, with the exception of low-carb products with 3 grams of Net Carbs or less.
- Any food made with added sugar of any sort, including but not limited to pastries, cookies, cakes, and candy. (See "The Scoop on Sugar: Fat Took the Hit for Sugar," on page 10.)
- Alcohol in any form.
- Nuts and seeds, nut and seed butters, and nut flours or meals, with the exception of flax meal and coconut flour. (Nuts and seeds are okay after two weeks in Phase 1.)
- Grains, even whole grains.
- Kidney beans, chickpeas, lentils, and other legumes.
- Starchy vegetables such as carrots, potatoes, sweet potatoes, and winter squash. Check the Atkins Carb Counter if you're unsure.
- Dairy products other than cream, sour cream, half-and-half, and aged cheeses. No cow or goat milk, yogurt, cottage cheese, or ricotta for now.
- "Low-fat" foods, which are usually higher in carbs.
- "Diet" products, unless they specifically state "low carbohydrate" and have no more than 3 grams of Net Carbs per serving.
- "Junk food" in any form.
- Products such as chewing gum, breath mints, cough syrups and drops, or liquid vitamins, unless they're sweetened with sorbitol

or xylitol. You can have up to three a day of those. Count 1 gram
per piece.

You may want to photocopy this list and place it on your refrigerator door.

WEEK-AT-A-GLANCE WEEK 1 MEAL PLANS

To make things as easy as possible, I've prepared two simple meal plans
to follow in your first week, along with shopping lists of everything
you'll need. The meal plan on page 62 includes Atkins products; the
one on page 64 does not. You'll be eating protein, foundation vegetables, and acceptable Phase 1 (Kick-Start) dairy products, as illustrated
on the first rung of the Carb Ladder (page 16).

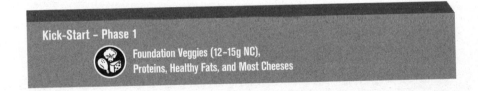

Kick-Start – Phase 1
Foundation Veggies (12–15g NC),
Proteins, Healthy Fats, and Most Cheeses

Of course, you can modify either meal plan to suit your preferences
as long as you stay within the Phase 1 acceptable foods guidelines. For
example:

- If you don't eat red meat, simply substitute fish, shellfish, poultry, or tofu for pork, beef, etc.
- If you prefer other foundation veggies, sub them in for those
  listed.
- You can swap one or more items with a recipe from the recipe
  section (page 245) or the online recipe database.

Atkins Phase 1 (Kick-Start) Meal Plan at 20g NC/day: Week 1

	Monday	Tuesday	Wednesday	Thursday
BREAKFAST	2 eggs ¼ cup chopped onion 1 tsp olive oil 1 oz Cheddar cheese 2 oz bacon or sausage **Net Carbs: 4.1g; FV: 3.1g**	Atkins Advantage Peanut Butter Granola Bar **Net Carbs: 3g; FV: 0g**	Atkins Frozen Farmhouse-Style Sausage Scramble **Net Carbs: 5g; FV: 1g**	4–6 oz steak or hamburger 1 tsp olive oil ½ cup chopped bell pepper ¼ cup chopped onion 2 oz Cheddar cheese **Net Carbs: 6g; FV: 5.3g**
SNACK	Atkins Advantage Vanilla Shake **Net Carbs: 1g; FV: 0g**	1 small tomato 2 oz Monterey Jack cheese **Net Carbs: 2.8g; FV: 2.5g**	¾ cup sliced bell pepper 2 Tbsp ranch dressing **Net Carbs: 3.5g; FV: 2.8g**	Atkins Advantage Milk Chocolate Delight Shake **Net Carbs: 2g; FV: 0g**
LUNCH	Atkins Frozen Crustless Chicken Pot Pie **Net Carbs: 5g; FV: 4g**	4–6 oz chicken 1 small tomato 1 cup mixed greens ½ avocado 2 Tbsp ranch dressing **Net Carbs: 5.8g; FV: 5.1g**	Atkins Frozen Beef Merlot **Net Carbs: 6g; FV: 4g**	4–6 oz ham or pork chop 1 cup baby spinach ½ avocado 2 Tbsp ranch dressing* **Net Carbs: 3.9g; FV: 2.8g**
SNACK	Atkins Advantage Coconut Almond Delight Bar **Net Carbs: 3g; FV: 0g**	1 stalk celery 2 oz Cheddar cheese **Net Carbs: 1.7g; FV: 1g**	Atkins Advantage Café Caramel Shake **Net Carbs: 2g; FV: 0g**	1 small tomato 2 Tbsp vinaigrette **Net Carbs: 2.9g; FV: 2.5g**
DINNER	4–6 oz canned tuna or fish filet 2 cups mixed greens ½ avocado 2 Tbsp vinaigrette 1 cup broccoli florets 1 Tbsp butter **Net Carbs: 6g; FV: 5.6g**	Atkins Frozen Meatloaf with Portobello Mushroom Gravy **Net Carbs: 7g; FV: 4g**	4–6 oz chicken 1 cup broccoli florets 1 Tbsp olive oil 2 cups mixed greens 2 Tbsp creamy Italian dressing **Net Carbs: 4.5g; FV: 4.3g**	Atkins Frozen Chicken and Broccoli Alfredo **Net Carbs: 5g; FV: 5g**
	Total Net Carbs: 19.1g **Total Net Carbs from FV: 12.7g**	**Total Net Carbs: 20.3g** **Total Net Carbs from FV: 12.6g**	**Total Net Carbs: 21g** **Total Net Carbs from FV: 12.1g**	**Total Net Carbs: 19.8g** **Total Net Carbs from FV: 15.6g**

Enjoy Atkins Endulge Treats for dessert if Net Carb consumption allows!

Friday	Saturday	Sunday
1 cup baby spinach 1 small tomato ½ avocado 1 oz Monterey Jack cheese	Atkins Frozen Tex-Mex Scramble	2 eggs 2 cups baby spinach 1 Tbsp olive oil ½ bell pepper 2 oz Monterey Jack cheese
Net Carbs: 5.3g; FV: 5.3g	**Net Carbs: 5g; FV: 3g**	**Net Carbs: 6.4g; FV: 5.3g**
2 oz Cheddar cheese 1 small tomato 2 Tbsp vinaigrette	Atkins Advantage Caramel Chocolate Nut Roll Bar	1 stalk celery 2 oz Cheddar cheese
Net Carbs: 3.6g; FV: 2.5g	**Net Carbs: 3g; FV: 0g**	**Net Carbs: 1.7g; FV: 1g**
Atkins Frozen Roast Turkey Tenders with Herb Pan Gravy	4–6 oz canned tuna or fish filet 2 Tbsp mayonnaise or tartar sauce 1 stalk celery ¼ cup chopped bell pepper 1 small tomato	Atkins Advantage Chocolate Peanut Butter Bar
Net Carbs: 6g; FV: 4g	**Net Carbs: 5g; FV: 5g**	**Net Carbs: 2g; FV: 0g**
Atkins Advantage Caramel Chocolate Peanut Nougat Bar	Atkins Advantage Vanilla Shake	½ cup chopped bell pepper 2 Tbsp ranch dressing
Net Carbs: 3g; FV: 0g	**Net Carbs: 1g; FV: 0g**	**Net Carbs: 2.9g; FV: 2.2g**
4–6 oz ham or pork chop 1 cup broccoli 1 Tbsp butter 1 cup mixed greens 2 Tbsp creamy Italian dressing	4–6 oz steak or hamburger 1 oz Cheddar cheese 1 small tomato ½ avocado ½ small onion, sliced	Atkins Frozen Crustless Chicken Pot Pie
Net Carbs: 3.2g; FV: 2.9g	**Net Carbs: 6.7g; FV: 6.5g**	**Net Carbs: 5g; FV: 4g**
Total Net Carbs: 21.1g **Total Net Carbs from** **FV: 14.7g**	**Total Net Carbs: 20.7g** **Total Net Carbs from** **FV: 14.5g**	**Total Net Carbs: 18g** **Total Net Carbs from** **FV: 12.5g**

Atkins Phase 1 (Kick-Start) Meal Plan at 20g NC/day: Week 1 (no Atkins products)

	Monday	Tuesday	Wednesday	Thursday

BREAKFAST	2 eggs
	¼ cup chopped onion
	1 tsp olive oil
	1 oz Cheddar cheese
	2 oz bacon or sausage
	
	Net Carbs: 4.1g; FV: 3.1g
		4–6 oz bacon or sausage
		½ cup chopped bell
		   pepper
		
		Net Carbs: 3g; FV: 2.2g
			2 eggs
			2–4 oz ham or pork chop
			1 Tbsp olive oil
			3 Tbsp chopped onion
			½ small tomato
			
			Net Carbs: 4.6g; FV: 3.5g
				4–6 oz steak or hamburger
				1 tsp olive oil
				½ cup chopped bell
				   pepper
				¼ cup chopped onion
				2 oz Cheddar cheese
				Net Carbs: 6g; FV: 5.3g

SNACK	2 stalks celery
	2 Tbsp creamy Italian
	   dressing
	Net Carbs: 2.2g; FV: 2g
		1 small tomato
		2 oz Monterey Jack
		   cheese
		Net Carbs: 2.8g; FV: 2.5g
			¾ cup sliced bell pepper
			2 Tbsp ranch dressing
			
			Net Carbs: 3.5g; FV: 2.8g
				1 stalk celery
				1 oz mozzarella cheese
				
				Net Carbs: 1.2g; FV: 1g

LUNCH	4–6 oz ham or
	   pork chop
	1 small tomato
	1 cup baby spinach
	2 Tbsp vinaigrette
	
	Net Carbs: 4.3g; FV: 4g
		4–6 oz chicken
		1 small tomato
		1 cup mixed greens
		½ avocado
		2 Tbsp ranch dressing
		
		Net Carbs: 5.8g; FV: 5.1g
			4–6 oz steak or
			   hamburger
			1 cup mixed greens
			½ avocado
			2 Tbsp vinaigrette
			
			Net Carbs: 3g; FV: 2.6g
				4–6 oz ham or
				   pork chop
				1 cup baby spinach
				½ avocado
				2 Tbsp ranch dressing
				
				Net Carbs: 3.9g; FV: 2.8g

SNACK	½ cup sliced bell pepper 2 Tbsp ranch dressing **Net Carbs: 2.6g; FV: 1.8g**	1 stalk celery 2 oz Cheddar cheese **Net Carbs: 1.7g; FV: 1g**	1 small tomato 1 oz Monterey Jack cheese **Net Carbs: 2.6g; FV: 2.5g**	1 small tomato 2 Tbsp vinaigrette **Net Carbs: 2.9g; FV: 2.5g**

DINNER	4–6 oz canned tuna or
	   fish filet
	2 cups mixed greens
	½ avocado
	2 Tbsp vinaigrette
	1 cup broccoli florets
	1 Tbsp butter
	Net Carbs: 6g; FV: 5.6g
		4–6 oz steak or hamburger
		½ medium bell pepper
		⅓ small onion
		1 Tbsp olive oil
		1 cup mixed greens
		2 Tbsp ranch dressing
		
		Net Carbs: 6.3g; FV: 5.5g
			4–6 oz chicken
			1 cup broccoli florets
			1 Tbsp olive oil
			2 cups mixed greens
			2 Tbsp creamy Italian
			   dressing
			
			Net Carbs: 4.5g; FV: 4.3g
				4–6 oz chicken
				2 cups baby spinach
				½ cup sliced bell pepper
				1 small tomato
				2 Tbsp ranch dressing
				
				Net Carbs: 6.5g; FV: 5.8g

	Total Net Carbs: 19.2g
	Total Net Carbs from
	   FV: 16.5g
		Total Net Carbs: 19.6g
		Total Net Carbs from
		   FV: 16.3g
			Total Net Carbs: 18.2g
			Total Net Carbs from
			   FV: 15.7g
				Total Net Carbs: 20.5g
				Total Net Carbs from
				   FV: 17.4g

Enjoy Atkins Endulge Treats for dessert if Net Carb consumption allows!

Friday	Saturday	Sunday

1 cup baby spinach
1 small tomato
½ avocado
1 oz Monterey Jack
  cheese
	2 eggs
	2 oz bacon or sausage
	1 small tomato
		2 eggs
		2 cups baby spinach
		1 Tbsp olive oil
		½ of 1 bell pepper
		2 oz Monterey Jack
		  cheese

Net Carbs: 5.3g; FV: 5.3g	**Net Carbs: 4.5g; FV: 2.5g**	**Net Carbs: 6.4g; FV: 5.3g**
2 oz Cheddar cheese 1 small tomato 2 Tbsp vinaigrette	½ cup sliced bell pepper 2 oz Monterey Jack cheese	1 stalk celery 2 oz Cheddar cheese
Net Carbs: 3.6g; FV: 2.5g	**Net Carbs: 2.2g; FV: 1.8g**	**Net Carbs: 1.7g; FV: 1g**

4–6 oz chicken
2 cups mixed greens
½ cup sliced bell
  pepper
2 Tbsp creamy Italian
  dressing
	4–6 oz canned tuna or
	  fish filet
	2 Tbsp mayonnaise or
	  tartar sauce
	1 stalk celery
	¼ cup chopped bell
	  pepper
	1 small tomato
		4–6 oz ham or pork
		2 cups baby spinach
		1 medium tomato
		2 Tbsp vinaigrette

Net Carbs: 4.8g; FV: 4.5g	**Net Carbs: 5g; FV: 5g**	**Net Carbs: 5.6g; FV: 4.8g**

2 stalks celery
2 oz Cheddar cheese
	½ avocado
	2 ½ Tbsp creamy Italian
	  dressing
		½ cup chopped bell
		  pepper
		2 Tbsp ranch dressing

Net Carbs: 2.7g; FV: 2g	**Net Carbs: 1.5g; FV: 1.3g**	**Net Carbs: 2.9g; FV: 2.2g**

4–6 oz ham or pork
  chop
1 cup broccoli
1 cup mixed greens
2 Tbsp creamy Italian
  dressing
	4–6 oz steak or
	  hamburger
	1 oz Cheddar cheese
	1 small tomato
	½ avocado
	½ small onion, sliced
		6 oz chicken
		1 cup broccoli
		1 Tbsp olive oil
		1 cup mixed greens
		½ avocado
		2 Tbsp vinaigrette

Net Carbs: 3.2g; FV: 2.9g	**Net Carbs: 6.7g; FV: 6.5g**	**Net Carbs: 4.6g; FV: 4.2g**
Total Net Carbs: 19.6g **Total Net Carbs from** ** FV: 17.2g**	**Total Net Carbs: 19.9g** **Total Net Carbs from** ** FV: 17.1g**	**Total Net Carbs: 21.2g** **Total Net Carbs from** ** FV: 17.5g**

WEEK 1 SHOPPING LIST

Assuming you follow the meal plan to the letter, this short shopping list enables you to have everything at hand to get a week's worth of meals on the table. If you're not using Atkins products, simply adjust the list. Likewise, if you modify the meal plan, you'll need to make comparable changes to the shopping list.

WEEK 1

PROTEINS	DAIRY/CHEESE	VEGETABLES	SAUCES/CONDIMENTS	ATKINS PRODUCTS
Steak or Hamburgers	Butter	Hass Avocados	Creamy Italian Dressing*	Atkins Bars
Chicken	Cheddar Cheese	Baby Spinach	Mayonnaise* or Tartar Sauce*	Atkins Shakes
Eggs	Monterey Jack Cheese	Broccoli Florets	Ranch Dressing*	Atkins Frozen Meals
Ham or Pork Chops		Celery	Vinaigrette*	
Canned Tuna or Fish Filets		Lettuce/ Mixed Greens	Extra Virgin Olive Oil	
Bacon or Sausages		Onions		
		Green or Red Bell Peppers		
		Tomatoes		

*Select sauces and condiments without added sugar.

The first meal plan incorporates a number of Atkins frozen meals, as well as our bars and shakes. It requires only twenty-four common ingredients, a number of which you probably already have in your fridge, pantry, or freezer, saving you time both shopping and cooking. The second meal plan includes more made-from-scratch meals and therefore more ingredients. You can also mix the two plans, relying on more Atkins frozen meals on days when time is at a premium or substituting Atkins bars or shakes for snacks or breakfast when you're on the run.

Both plans indicate the number of grams of Net Carbs from foundation vegetables, making it easy to ensure that you're getting enough of these nutritious and filling carbohydrate foods. Neither plan includes beverages; add grams of Net Carbs in cream, lighteners, or sweeteners in beverages to your daily tally.

If you're creating your own meal plans, be sure to spread your carb intake out across the day to keep your blood sugar on an even keel. Aim for roughly 3–5 grams of Net Carbs at breakfast, 5–7 at lunch, and the same at dinner. Snacks can range from 1 to 3 grams.

A GAME PLAN FOR MEALS AWAY FROM HOME

If you work outside the home, you're likely to eat out at least once a day. So give some thought to how you're going to find low-carb meals and snacks on those occasions. Think about what your typical day looks like now.

- Which meals do you eat at home?
- Which do you bring to work with you?
- Which do you order out?
- How often do you eat out?
- Do you take coffee breaks or keep snack foods in your desk or locker?
- Do you often find yourself in airports and on planes, driving in areas devoid of good food choices, or just sitting in traffic?

Then think about what you actually eat at those times. If you typically grab a bagel on the way to work, eat lunch—usually a sandwich—out, and often order pizza for dinner on weeknights, just stocking your kitchen with Atkins-friendly foods won't address all your needs.

- Keep some Atkins frozen meals in the freezer at work and use the shakes and bars for a convenient, on-the-go breakfast or snack.
- Check out possibilities online, where most eateries post their menus, or with your Atkins mobile app, using the Dining Out feature.
- Find a diner or deli where you can pick up scrambled eggs or another suitable breakfast.
- Check out the nearest salad bar for good lunch choices.
- Come up with takeout places or restaurants that deliver for dinner.

With your away-from-home meal sources identified and the right items in your pantry, you'll be good to go. (For more on eating outside the home, see Chapter 10, "Dine Out with Ease.")

STOP CERTAIN SYMPTOMS BEFORE THEY START

A few small changes in your routine can help you avoid some unpleasant (and absolutely unnecessary) symptoms that could occur in the first couple of weeks as your body converts to a fat-burning machine. That's when some people experience fatigue, weakness, constipation, headaches, or leg cramps. Or light-headedness can occur when rising too quickly from a seated position, stepping out of a hot shower or hot tub, or simply engaging in household chores on a hot summer day. Some people complain that they feel "brain fog." Others refer to it as "Atkins flu."

These symptoms have nothing to do with eating fewer carbs or more protein and fat. Instead, they are the result of a deficit of sodium (salt). Eating the low-carb way is naturally diuretic. That's why you quickly lose those water pounds that can make you look bloated and puffy. Along with water, sodium and other minerals called electrolytes are flushed from your body. Just as an athlete needs to rehydrate and replace lost electrolytes when perspiring profusely, it's essential that you drink plenty of liquids and consume adequate salt to replace the water and sodium you're losing.

One of the reasons I emphasize eating a minimum amount of foundation vegetables each day is that they're full of both water and minerals, including sodium. They are also rich in fiber, which helps avoid constipation. But they may not contain enough sodium for you, especially if you've been eating a lot of salty snack foods until now or are fairly active. To ensure that you escape the above symptoms (or, at the very least, moderate them), I strongly suggest that you add a little extra sodium to your diet. (See "Sensitive to Salt?", below, if you have high blood pressure.) There are three ways you can do this. Each day, in addition to salting your food as you always have, add one of the following:

- An additional ½ teaspoon salt
- 2 tablespoons regular (not low-sodium) tamari (soy sauce)
- 2 cups regular (not low-sodium) beef, chicken, or vegetable broth—you can used the canned kind or a bouillon cube in boiling water

SENSITIVE TO SALT?

If you have hypertension and take diuretics to control your blood pressure, talk to your health care provider before adding additional sodium to your diet. Many people find that their blood pressure drops naturally when they start eating the low-carb way, so monitor your blood pressure when you start Atkins and discuss any change in dosage with him or her.

If you're experiencing any of the symptoms described above, you can add another 5 grams of Net Carbs in the form of nuts or seeds or a small can of tomato juice until you feel like yourself again. Then drop back to 20 grams of Net Carbs (and omit the nuts or tomato juice) to fast-track weight loss.

THE SCOOP ON SUGAR: MULTIPLE ALIASES

Like some criminals, sugar commits its offenses under many names. Regardless of the name, sugar in foods and beverages quickly turns to blood sugar (and then fat) in your body. Some names indicate the source of the sugar: cane, date, grape, maple, or beet sugar. Others indicate color: white, brown, yellow, or golden sugar. Some refer to texture: confectioners', superfine (castor), or icing sugar. Other names imply minimal processing: raw, Demerara, turbinado, or muscovado. Some are familiar: caramel, honey, maple syrup, or molasses. Bottom line: they're all sugar. Also be on the lookout for these aliases on the labels of packaged foods:

- Agave syrup or crystals
- Barley malt
- Cane juice crystals
- Corn syrup, corn syrup solids, high-fructose corn syrup
- Dextran or dextrose
- Diastase, diastatic malt
- Fructose
- Fruit juice, fruit juice concentrate
- Galactose
- Glucose, glucose solids
- Golden syrup
- Lactose
- Maltose, maltol
- Refiner's syrup
- Rice syrup
- Sorghum syrup
- Sucrose
- Treacle

FREQUENTLY ASKED QUESTIONS

Q. Do I have to start Atkins in Phase 1?

A. No. You can start in any of the first three phases. If you have just a few pounds to lose, up to about 15, you can probably start in Phase 2 (Balancing) at 25 to 30 grams of Net Carbs a day. If you are heavier, you can also start here, but it could take considerably longer to lose weight without the kick start that you get in Phase 1. You can also begin in Phase 3 (Fine-Tuning) at, say, 45 grams of Net Carbs a day if you have very little weight to lose or are willing to shed it very slowly.

Q. Do I have to count carbs if I follow the meal plans exactly?

A. No. However, it's unlikely that you'll follow them to the letter day in and day out unless you eat every meal at home, so it's a good idea to use the Atkins Carb Counter. Also, if you aren't precise about serving size, you may be consuming more carbs than the meal plan indicates. In any case, it's important to know how to count carbs (actually, grams of Net Carbs) as you start to add back more foods. Counting provides a double check that improves your likelihood of success from the start.

Q. Must I have two snacks a day?

A. Not necessarily. If you're having four or five small meals a day, you may not feel the need for snacks, but be very careful not to go more than four to six hours between meals. Instead, have a hot drink, perhaps a cup of broth.

Q. What is water weight loss?

A. The first few pounds you lose on any weight-loss program are primarily water, and Atkins has a particularly diuretic effect. That's why it's essential to drink plenty of water and other fluids, eat your foundation veggies, and take a multivitamin-mineral supplement to replace the electrolytes you'll be flushing out of your body along with the excess fluid. After the first few days you'll be losing primarily body fat.

Q. Can I eat as much protein and fat as I wish?

A. No. Eating excessive protein will make you sluggish and interfere with weight loss. Overeat fat and you'll burn it and not body fat for energy. Follow the guidelines on pages 57 and 58.

Q. Why do I have to drink so much water?

A. Most people are borderline dehydrated all the time. Drinking enough fluid helps flush toxins from your body, combats constipation and bad breath, lubricates your joints, and is important to your overall health. Staying hydrated also assists with weight loss. Remember, some of your water requirement can be satisfied with coffee, tea, or other clear beverages, including broth.

Q. Most bacon is sugar or maple cured. Does that mean I can't eat bacon?
A. Bacon is fine in moderation. Any residual sugar from the curing process in bacon, ham, or other pork products is burned off when you cook it.

Q. Why do the carb counts for some vegetables differ depending upon whether they're raw or cooked?
A. Cooking compacts vegetables such as spinach or cabbage significantly. Carb counts reflect the cooked amount. Chopping or grating a vegetable also compacts it more than slicing does, and that impacts the carb count as well.

Q. Can I have dessert in Phase 1?
A. Yes, as long as you get your quota of foundation vegetables and don't exceed your Net Carb daily limit. A dessert should contain no more than 3 grams of Net Carbs per serving. An Atkins Endulge bar or one of our dessert recipes is a good choice.

TIME TO EVALUATE YOUR PROGRESS

After seven days in Phase 1 (Kick-Start), weigh and measure yourself. If you've lost several pounds and inches, you've almost certainly lost fat in addition to the initial fluid loss. If you've lost only inches or more inches than pounds, don't worry. Inches often show up first and the pounds are sure to follow. Keep doing what you're doing!

What if you lost just a pound or two? That's still nothing to sneeze at. Check your measurements too. You may have made more progress there. And try to see the glass as half full. After all, you weigh less than you did a week ago. Also think about how your clothes are fitting. If you're disappointed with your rate of loss, ask yourself whether your expectations were reasonable. While some people can lose up to 15 pounds in two weeks, weight-loss patterns differ significantly from one person to another. And even if you could banish a pound a day when you were in your twenties, it's unlikely you can do so in your forties. On the other hand, the heavier you are, the more quickly you'll lose weight. Men usually lose faster than women, as do physically active people. Hormonal issues can make weight loss difficult.

If you're sure that you were doing everything by the book your first week on Atkins, take this dietary reality test:

1. *Are you counting grams of Net Carbs?* If you're just estimating or you're not taking serving size into consideration, there's a good chance you're overdoing the carbs and haven't kick-started your fat-burning engine. Use your Atkins Carb Counter and track in your journal everything you eat.

2. *Are you skipping meals or going too long without eating?* If so, you may get ravenous and overeat. Be sure to eat a meal or snack every three or four hours.

3. *Did you consume less than 18 or more than 22 grams of Net Carbs each day?* Having too few or too many carbs can interfere with jump-starting fat burning. See #1.

4. *Are you drinking eight glasses of acceptable liquids?* If not, increase your intake, using such tricks as setting the alarm on your cell phone or filling a quart container with water twice a day. Being dehydrated can slow fat burning and produce other unpleasant side effects.

5. *Did you eat a minimum of 12–15 grams of Net Carbs from foundation vegetables each day?* This is not negotiable for the reasons stated earlier. If you haven't been doing this, get with the program and you'll see the pounds start to melt away.

6. *Are you eating more than the recommended amount of protein?* Unless you're a very tall man, if you're eating more than 6 ounces of protein at a single meal, you're overdoing it. Review and follow the guidelines provided earlier in this chapter and weight loss should speed up.

7. *Are you holding back on fat?* Again, eating natural fats is essential to turn your body fat into your primary fuel source. Lose your fear of fat and lose your fat!

8. *Did you have more than three packets of sweetener a day?* Some people are more sensitive than others to sugar substitutes. Even the small amount of carbs in these products can interfere with weight loss in Phase 1. Cut down to half a packet for each serving, or omit them altogether for a week or two.

9. *Did you check the ingredients list of any packaged foods or condiments you ate?* If not, you may have unwittingly consumed some hidden sugars. Develop an eagle eye for reading labels!

10. *Are you taking any medications that could interfere with weight loss?* If so, review Chapter 2 and discuss with your physician.

If this checklist unearthed some misunderstandings about how to follow the program that are impeding your progress, simply make the recommended changes as you enter Week 2. If you haven't already done so, I can't overstate how important it is to keep a daily journal of what you eat. Doing so will allow you to quickly spot the problems cited above. Even small changes, such as using fewer packets of sweetener, can have a significant impact.

Now meet Mike D., who lost more than half his start weight and has kept it off for a decade. Then learn more about Phase 1 (Kick-Start) in Chapter 4. For starters, we'll look at ways to add variety to meals (especially breakfast), coordinate Atkins meals with family meals, and deal with some of the day-to-day challenges of getting meals on the table and in your tummy.

SUCCESS STORY

HALF THE MAN HE WAS,
AND BETTER FOR IT

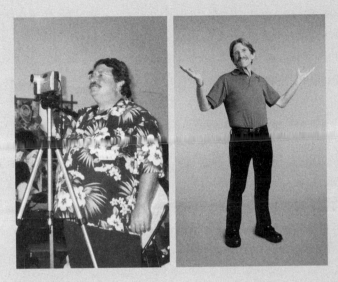

VITAL STATS

Daily Net Carb intake: 20–30
  grams
Age: 62
Height: 5'3"

Before weight: 300 pounds
After weight: 125 pounds
Weight lost: 175 pounds

In 2004 when audiovisual consultant Mike D., of Napa, California, told his physician he wanted gastric bypass surgery, he was informed that he first needed to lose 10 percent of his 300 pounds. After two months on Atkins and minus 30 pounds, Mike decided to see if he could lose more weight without going under the knife. It took him fourteen months to achieve that goal, and he's maintained his trim 125-pound transformation since then. Mike tells his story.

My wife and I renewed our marriage vows in Las Vegas in 2003 in front of an Elvis Presley impersonator. Our first wedding was in a grotto in Hawaii, but that wasn't the only difference. The second time I weighed more than twice what I did when we married fifteen years earlier! Now, as our twenty-fifth anniversary approaches, I'm back to the weight I was as a groom.

I wasn't into most sweets, but I really liked high-carb food like chips, dips, and pies. I used to make a cherry cheesecake to die for. My workplace was sociable and we'd have lots of potlucks and were all into desserts. I'd tried cutting back but nothing gave fast enough weight-loss results. When my HMO started paying for gastric bypass surgery, I decided I wanted the weight off once and for all. I knew that with my smoking—I had a pack-and-a-half to two-pack habit—and being overweight, I was likely to die before my time.

I looked at several weight-loss programs, decided on Atkins, and stayed on a modified form of Induction the whole fourteen months it took me to lose the extra weight. One thing that helped me stay the course was that I'd reward myself with a new Hawaiian shirt for every 10 pounds I lost. When I started doing Atkins I had a 60-inch waist and was wearing size 6X shirts. My waist is now half what it was and I now wear a small or medium.

My wife and I share the cooking. While I was losing I ate mostly meat and salads. The rest of the family would also have baked potatoes, pasta, breads, and the like. They were totally supportive about my doing Atkins. Later my wife lost the 35 pounds she wanted to lose on the program. She and I find it easy to eat out. For example, we'll order prime ribs at our favorite diner but skip the corn bread and order extra vegetables instead.

Basically, I eat meats, cheese, salads, and cooked vegetables. I especially like chef salads with ranch dressing. Nowadays, my treats are peanuts, sugar-free chocolate candy, and Atkins bars. I've also found a great brand of low-carb bread called MiRico. It's the first bread I've had in ten years. and occasionally I'll have it with no-sugar-added jam. I do the grocery shopping and read labels carefully.

I'm aware of my carb intake but don't count carbs anymore. I realize now that the real key to weight loss is not the number of calories consumed in a day but the amount of carbs. At first I thought that I was "dieting" and that after I'd lost weight I'd go back to eating the things I used to eat. But I've come to understand that to keep weight off, it has to be a lifestyle change. My food preferences have actually changed a lot and I feel healthier.

When I went back to my doctor after losing the weight, he was amazed. All my health markers were excellent. When I told him that I did it on Atkins, he was delighted it had worked. His parting words were, "I probably won't see much of you from now on."

Losing weight on Atkins and being successful in keeping it off long-term came in handy when it was time to give up my thirty-year smoking habit. I wish I could say my decision was personal, but my workplace instituted a no-smoking policy. So it was give it up or go off premises every time I took a cigarette break. I was concerned that I might regain weight after I stopped smoking, but fortunately, I haven't. I seem to be a permanently slim guy!

MAKE IT EASY

My advice to anyone with more than 100 pounds to lose is to stay on Phase 1 longer than two weeks. *—M.D.*

CHAPTER 4

YOUR SECOND WEEK ON ATKINS

You're now on your eighth day of eating the Atkins way and are probably off and running. Give yourself a pat on the back and flash a high
five! You've almost certainly shed some of that padding around your
middle—belly fat is the first to go on Atkins—meaning there's a little
less of you to love. Your real weight loss should pick up now that you're
losing only fat and not water weight. If you experienced fatigue for a
few days as you transitioned to burning mostly fat, chances are that
has vanished. Almost everyone reports a burst of energy by Week 2,
and many people feel a sense of exhilaration. Perhaps most amazing
of all, you're experiencing that marvelous sense of being in control of
your appetite. Life is good! Stick with Atkins and it's only going to get
better.

By now you know the guidelines for Phase 1 (Kick-Start) and have
a good understanding of what's on the menu for the first two weeks
(and perhaps longer). In this chapter I'll show you how to branch out
a bit with more options for breakfast, lunch, dinner, and snacks, including a complete meal plan for the week. We'll also delve deeper
into the details of daily life in this phase, such as how to integrate

Atkins into family meals, and address some challenges you may be already experiencing or anticipating. Time is at a premium for all of us, so I know you're looking for ways to eat nutritious low-carb meals and snacks with a minimum of effort. Resolving these and other important issues from the start will build your confidence in the program and strengthen your commitment to stay the course.

SOLVING THE BREAKFAST DILEMMA

Breakfast on Atkins can be the most dramatic change from your usual eating pattern. No wonder. Just compare the typical low-carb and low-fat breakfasts below. The latter contains the equivalent of 18 teaspoons sugar (approximately ⅓ cup), and that doesn't include a teaspoon or two of sugar in coffee or tea and jam or jelly on the toast. On the other hand, the low-carb breakfast of two eggs cooked with ½ cup chopped onion and 1 ounce Cheddar cheese in 1 teaspoon olive oil, and 2 ounces bacon or sausage contains just 4.2 grams of Net Carbs—the equivalent of a single teaspoon of sugar. (For more breakfast carb bombs, see "The Scoop on Sugar: Sweets for Breakfast" on page 83.)

TYPICAL LOW-CARB BREAKFAST
Western Omelet

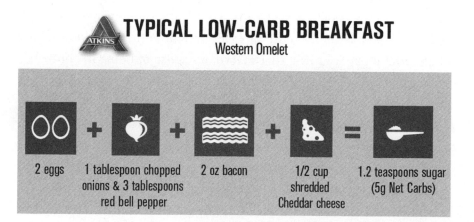

| 2 eggs | 1 tablespoon chopped onions & 3 tablespoons red bell pepper | 2 oz bacon | 1/2 cup shredded Cheddar cheese | 1.2 teaspoons sugar (5g Net Carbs) |

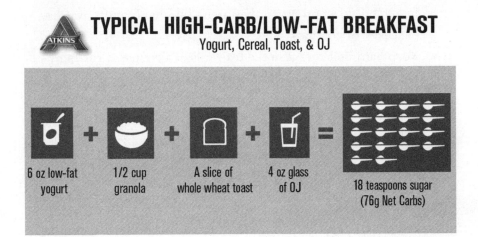

TYPICAL HIGH-CARB/LOW-FAT BREAKFAST
Yogurt, Cereal, Toast, & OJ

6 oz low-fat yogurt + 1/2 cup granola + A slice of whole wheat toast + 4 oz glass of OJ = 18 teaspoons sugar (76g Net Carbs)

There are a number of tasty and filling choices for breakfast in the first two weeks on Atkins. Let's start with the obvious. Egg lovers are in luck, as it's perfectly fine to have two or three eggs every day.

- Enjoy eggs poached, fried, scrambled, baked, hard-boiled, soft-boiled, or made into omelets or frittatas.
- Serve eggs with sliced tomato, grated cheese, a pat of goat cheese, bacon, sausage, or veggies (reheated leftovers are fine) such as cooked spinach, asparagus, or broccoli.
- Jazz them up with sugar-free salsa or guacamole.
- Try Eggs Parmesan (page 252) or Breakfast Casserole (page 255).
- Check out the Atkins recipe database for dozens more delectable egg dishes.

Okay, you like eggs. And they're great on the weekend when you can chill out, but not on rushed weekday mornings. Or there's no handy deli or coffee shop where you can pick up some scrambled eggs or an omelet—hold the toast—on your way to work. How about these ideas?

- Pop an Atkins Tex-Mex Scramble or Farmhouse Style Sausage Scramble frozen meal into the microwave. Unlike most other frozen breakfast products, they aren't built on biscuits, waffles, pancakes, or potatoes.

- Keep hard-boiled eggs in the fridge. Peel a couple in the morning, slice in half, and drizzle with hot sauce or top with a little mayo and salt and pepper. Or have one plus an Atkins shake or bar. No time to eat at home? What could be more portable than a hard-boiled egg neatly packaged in its shell?
- Make deviled eggs the night before, flavoring them with curry powder, pesto, chopped chives, or dill.
- Make a crustless quiche, dividing the mixture into six portions and cook in muffin tins. After they're cooled, freeze in individual portions and then reheat in the oven or microwave.
- No time to even boil eggs? You can find peeled, hard-boiled eggs in the dairy section of your supermarket, or at a salad bar, along with crumbled bacon.

EGGLESS BREAKFAST OPTIONS

Even confirmed egg-lovers have days when they simply want something else. Or perhaps even on a good day an egg is the last thing you want to see on your plate in the morning. What to do?

- Grab a tasty and convenient Atkins Day Break bar or shake.
- Check out the Atkins recipe database for Breakfast Mexi Peppers, Chicken-Portobello Broilers, Veggie Breakfast Sausage Stacked with Avocado and "Cheddar," and other tempting egg-free breakfast options.
- Breakfast sausage (or turkey or soy-based versions such as Gimme Lean) makes a hearty breakfast that cooks up fast. Stuff into portobello mushroom caps and broil. Or broil the sausage, stack with slices of mozzarella and tomato, and run under the broiler again.
- Pan-fried Canadian bacon also makes great breakfast stacks. How about one made with Cheddar cheese and salsa on the side?

THE SCOOP ON SUGAR: SWEETS FOR BREAKFAST

The typical American breakfast is made with white flour and sugar. In cereals the sugar may be in the form of dehydrated berries, marshmallows, honey, or maple syrup, adding to the already high carb count of grains. Hot cereals are right up there as well, particularly packaged ones. Orange juice might as well be liquid sugar, and bananas are among the fruits highest in carbs. Bagels are outta sight! Take a look at the carb minefield represented by a few breakfast faves:

SERVING	ITEM	NET CARBS (GRAMS)
1 packet	Instant cinnamon oatmeal	33
1 cup	Corn Chex	24
1 cup	Banana Nut Cheerios	22
½ cup	Grape-Nuts	27
½ cup	Alpen	38
½ cup	Bear Naked Maple Pecan Granola	40
1 cup	Frosted Mini-Wheats	40
½ cup	Orange juice	12
1 cup	Nonfat milk	10
3½-inch	Plain bagel	54
1	Strawberry Frosted Pop-Tart	35
2	Eggo Frozen Waffles	27
2 slices	White bread	24
1 small	Banana	20

- Pan-fry a skirt, minute, or other small steak and serve with veggie leftovers.
- Roll up sliced ham or another meat and/or cheese and a few other ingredients for a quick, satisfying, and portable breakfast. (See "Design a Roll-Up" on page 86, for more options.)
- Whip up a breakfast smoothie in no time in a blender, using sugar-free protein powder and unsweetened, unflavored almond milk, soy milk, or coconut milk beverage. Add sugar-free cocoa

powder or syrup and/or instant coffee granules. You can even hide some raw spinach or another leafy green in the mix. Pop in some ice cubes for a great frothy texture.

- Enjoy waffles and pancakes made with soy flour, flax meal, or coconut flour. Okay, pancakes and waffles are made with eggs, but I've never heard anyone turn them down for that reason! Check out Zucchini–Pumpkin Spice Pancakes (page 251) and Chocolate Waffles (page 253), and Buttermilk Cinnamon Waffles and Orange–Sour Cream Waffles (hold the Fresh Blueberry Sauce until you move to Phase 2) on atkins.com. You can make waffles or pancakes on the weekend, freeze, and then defrost in a toaster oven for speedy weekday breakfasts.

Frozen fully cooked pork or turkey bacon or sausages save time and minimize cleanup since most of the grease has been removed. Bacon comes in strips, Canadian-style rounds, or bits; sausage can be found as crumbles, patties, and links. Some frozen omelets are also available, but do check the ingredient list and Nutrition Facts panel to ensure they contain no added sugars or other unacceptable ingredients. Avoid bacon and sausage products cured with nitrates.

MAKE BREAKFAST AHEAD OF TIME

Many of the breakfast recipes on atkins.com and several of those in this book are ideal candidates for making in quantity and freezing in individual portions. For best results, keep the following in mind:

- If you're baking in muffin tins instead of a pie pan, reduce the oven temp by 25 degrees or so and the cooking time by 15 minutes and check for doneness at that point.
- Let quiches, muffins, and other baked goods come to room temperature before wrapping in plastic wrap and then aluminum foil and freezing for up to three months. Label and date each package.

- Remove the item the night before and let it defrost in the fridge, to reduce reheating time the next morning in a microwave or toaster oven.

LUNCH AND DINNER ON THE DOUBLE

The midday meal isn't the major hurdle that breakfast can be for most Atkins beginners. The simplest choice is an Atkins frozen meal—they're formulated to make it easy for you to stay on the plan. To reduce the carbs in most traditional lunch choices:

- Instead of, say, a turkey club sandwich, ditch the bread and order a big salad topped with sliced turkey.
- Or have several roll-ups—they're as portable as a sandwich—using sandwich components minus the bread (see "Design a Roll-Up" on page 86). Your turkey club could morph into a roll-up of slices of turkey filled with cheese, shredded lettuce, and sliced tomato. Yum!
- Deconstruct a cheeseburger or burger (toss the bun) and accompany it with a side salad. Some burger places now offer burgers wrapped in lettuce leaves.
- Any main-dish salad with 4–6 ounces of protein in the form of meat, poultry, fish, or shellfish makes a great lunch that can be prepared in minutes. If you put one together at a salad bar, be sure to pass on the chow mein noodles, raisins, corn relish, and other high-carb offerings. Our recipe developer has come up with five salad zingers, starting on page 270, suitable for all phases of Atkins. Also check atkins.com for more main dish salads.

If a salad leaves you wanting a little something more, a cup of hot broth may do the trick, as would any soup made with foundation veggies and/or protein, but minus noodles, rice, potatoes, or other starchy veggies. A smaller salad and a light soup such as Cream of Brocco-flower Soup (page 278) make a great combo too. A hearty soup, chowder, or stew such as No-Bean Chicken Chili (page 279), Taco Soup (page 280), or Salmon Mushroom Chowder (page 283) makes a complete lunch. There are plenty more delicious main-dish soups in the Atkins recipe database.

When ordering soup in a restaurant, ask about the ingredients. Many places use flour or cornstarch as a thickener and often sugar for flavor. Likewise, check the ingredients list in canned or packaged soups. The Atkins Carb Counter lists a few acceptable choices.

Dinner is actually the easiest meal to deal with as you move away from the standard American diet full of carbs. Rely on Atkins frozen meals on hectic evenings. When cooking from scratch, simply replace the potato, pasta, or rice you used to have with a second veggie serving or salad alongside your protein choice. You'll find lots more ways to make meals easier in Part III, "It's All About Food."

DESIGN A ROLL-UP

Mix and match the ingredients below to put together your own combinations. Feel free to combine cheese and meat as wraps. (You can also double-wrap in a lettuce leaf.) Three or four roll-ups make a great no-cook breakfast or lunch. One would serve as a super snack.

WRAPS	SPREADS	CENTERS
Sliced ham	Aioli	Asparagus
Sliced roast beef	Mayonnaise	Cucumber
Sliced turkey breast	Mustard	Avocado
Sliced smoked salmon	Cream cheese	Jicama
Swiss cheese	Soft goat cheese	Daikon
Monterey Jack	Egg salad	Roasted red pepper
Muenster cheese	Pickle slices or a gherkin	
Provolone		
Prosciutto		

PHASE 1 SNACKS PDQ

In addition to an Atkins Advantage shake or bar coded for Phase 1, the five snacks in the recipe section, and the old Atkins standbys of olives, half a Hass avocado, jerky (cured without sugar or nitrates), and pork rinds, here are some easy and satisfying alternatives. None contains more than 3 grams of Net Carbs per serving.

- A serving of bell pepper or zucchini slices, cherry tomatoes, radishes, or almost any raw foundation vegetable with 1 tablespoon ranch, blue cheese, Italian, or other low-carb dressing
- An ounce of string cheese
- Celery stuffed with salmon cream cheese
- Cucumber "boat" filled with tuna salad
- A lettuce leaf wrapped around grated Cheddar
- Shrimp cocktail with no-sugar-added cocktail sauce such as Trinity Hill Farms or Walden Farms
- Two slices of tomato topped with chopped fresh basil and grated mozzarella and run under the broiler for a minute

WEEK-AT-A-GLANCE MEAL 2 MEAL PLANS

Here's another week's worth of delicious, easy-to-prepare meals suitable for Phase 1 (Kick-Start), one with Atkins products and one without. You'll continue to follow the first rung on the Carb Ladder (page 16), eating protein, foundation vegetables, and acceptable Phase 1 dairy products. Review the suggestions in this chapter for modifying the Week 1 meal plan with recipes in this book and the online database. Or substitute any meal suggestion from the earlier meal plan. The shopping list for this week's plan (page 92) includes only six new items, which appear in boldface italics. You'll also need to replenish your supplies of fresh foods and perhaps some other items. Be sure to adjust your shopping list if you've modified the meal plan.

Atkins Phase 1 (Kick-Start) Meal Plan at 20g NC/day: Week 2

	Monday	Tuesday	Wednesday	Thursday
BREAKFAST	Atkins Advantage Chocolate Chip Granola Bar	Atkins Frozen Farmhouse-Style Sausage Scramble	2 eggs ¼ cup chopped bell pepper ½ avocado 1 oz pepper Jack cheese ⅛ cup salsa	Atkins Advantage Strawberry Almond Bar
	Net Carbs: 3g; FV: 0g	**Net Carbs: 5g; FV: 1g**	**Net Carbs: 5.7g; FV: 4g**	**Net Carbs: 3g; FV: 0g**
SNACK	½ avocado 2 Tbsp ranch dressing	1 cup sliced bell pepper 2 Tbsp blue cheese dressing	Atkins Advantage Vanilla Shake	1 stalk celery 2 oz Cheddar cheese
	Net Carbs: 2g; FV: 1.3g	**Net Carbs: 3.4g; FV: 2.7g**	**Net Carbs: 1g; FV: 0g**	**Net Carbs: 1.7g; FV: 1g**
LUNCH	Atkins Frozen Chicken Marsala	Atkins Frozen Beef Merlot	4–6 oz ham or pork chop 1 cup mixed greens ½ small tomato 2 Tbsp blue cheese dressing	Atkins Frozen Chicken and Broccoli Alfredo
	Net Carbs: 7g; FV: 3g	**Net Carbs: 6g; FV: 4g**	**Net Carbs: 3.7g; FV: 2.6g**	**Net Carbs: 5g; FV: 5g**
SNACK	1 medium tomato 2 oz pepper Jack cheese	Atkins Advantage Milk Chocolate Delight Shake	½ cup sliced bell pepper 2 Tbsp ranch dressing	Atkins Advantage Café Caramel Shake
	Net Carbs: 5.3g; FV: 3.3g	**Net Carbs: 2g; FV: 0g**	**Net Carbs: 2.6g; FV: 1.9g**	**Net Carbs: 2g; FV: 0g**
DINNER	Atkins Frozen Crustless Chicken Pot Pie	4–6 oz canned tuna or fish filet 1 cup mixed greens ½ avocado 1½ oz mozzarella cheese 2 Tbsp creamy Italian dressing ½ cup green beans 1 Tbsp butter	Atkins Frozen Roast Turkey Tenders with Herb Pan Gravy	4–6 oz ham or pork chop 1 cup cauliflower florets 1 oz Cheddar cheese 2 cups mixed greens 2 Tbsp ranch dressing
	Net Carbs: 5g; FV: 4g	**Net Carbs: 5g; FV: 4.7g**	**Net Carbs: 6g; FV: 4g**	**Net Carbs: 7g; FV: 5.9g**
	Total Net Carbs: 22.3g **Total Net Carbs from FV: 11.6g**	**Total Net Carbs: 21.4g** **Total Net Carbs from FV: 12.4g**	**Total Net Carbs: 19g** **Total Net Carbs from FV: 12.5g**	**Total Net Carbs: 18.7g** **Total Net Carbs from FV: 11.9g**

Enjoy Atkins Endulge Treats for dessert if Net Carb consumption allows!

Friday	Saturday	Sunday
Atkins Frozen Tex-Mex Scramble	2 small tomatoes 4 oz bacon or sausage 1 oz Cheddar cheese	Atkins Frozen Farmhouse-Style Sausage Scramble
Net Carbs: 5g; FV: 3g	**Net Carbs: 5.3g; FV: 4.9g**	**Net Carbs: 5g; FV: 1g**
Atkins Day Break Cranberry Almond Bar	½ cup sliced bell pepper 2 Tbsp ranch dressing	Atkins Advantage Mocha Latte Shake
Net Carbs: 2g; FV: 0g	**Net Carbs: 2.6g; FV: 1.9g**	**Net Carbs: 2g; FV: 0g**
4–6 oz canned tuna or fish filet 2 Tbsp mayonnaise or tartar sauce 1½ stalks celery 3 cups mixed greens ½ avocado 2 Tbsp creamy Italian dressing	Atkins Advantage Chocolate Peanut Butter Bar	4–6 oz steak or hamburger 1 cup mixed greens 1 small tomato ½ cup sliced bell pepper ½ avocado 2 Tbsp vinaigrette
Net Carbs: 7g; FV: 6.9g	**Net Carbs: 2g; FV: 0g**	**Net Carbs: 6.8g; FV: 6.5g**
Atkins Strawberry Shake	1 small tomato 2 oz mozzarella cheese	Atkins Advantage Caramel Chocolate Peanut Nougat Bar
Net Carbs: 1g; FV: 0g	**Net Carbs: 2.5g; FV: 2.5g**	**Net Carbs: 3g; FV: 0g**
Atkins Frozen Sesame Chicken Stir-Fry	4–6 oz steak or hamburger ½ cup green beans 1 Tbsp olive oil 1 cup mixed greens ½ avocado 2 Tbsp blue cheese dressing	4–6 oz chicken 1 cup cauliflower florets 1 Tbsp butter 1 cup mixed greens 2 Tbsp creamy Italian dressing
Net Carbs: 7g; FV: 2g	**Net Carbs: 5.4g; FV: 4.7g**	**Net Carbs: 4.8g; FV: 4.5g**
Total Net Carbs: 22g **Total Net Carbs from FV: 11.9g**	**Total Net Carbs: 17.8g** **Total Net Carbs from FV: 14g**	**Total Net Carbs: 21.6g** **Total Net Carbs from FV: 12g**

Atkins Phase 1 (Kick-Start) Meal Plan at 20g NC/day: Week 2 (no Atkins products)

	Monday	Tuesday	Wednesday	Thursday
BREAKFAST	2 eggs ½ cup chopped bell pepper 1 oz mozzarella cheese 4 oz bacon or sausage **Net Carbs: 2.9g; FV: 2.2g**	1 small tomato ½ avocado 2 oz bacon or sausage 1 oz pepper Jack cheese **Net Carbs: 4.7g; FV: 3.8g**	2 eggs ¼ cup chopped bell pepper ½ avocado 1 oz pepper Jack cheese ⅛ cup salsa **Net Carbs: 5.7g; FV: 4g**	2 oz bacon or sausage ½ cup chopped bell pepper ¼ cup chopped onion 1 oz Cheddar cheese **Net Carbs: 5.6g; FV: 5.3g**
SNACK	½ avocado 2 Tbsp ranch dressing **Net Carbs: 2g; FV: 1.3g**	1 cup sliced bell pepper 2 Tbsp blue cheese dressing **Net Carbs: 3.4g; FV: 2.7g**	1 small tomato 1 oz mozzarella cheese **Net Carbs: 2.5g; FV: 2.5g**	1 stalk celery 2 oz Cheddar cheese **Net Carbs: 1.7g; FV: 1g**
LUNCH	4–6 oz chicken 1 small tomato 1 cup mixed greens 2 Tbsp blue cheese dressing **Net Carbs: 4.6g; FV: 3.8g**	4–6 oz steak or hamburger 1 cup mixed greens 2 Tbsp ranch dressing **Net Carbs: 2.1g; FV: 1.3g**	4–6 oz ham or pork chop 1 cup mixed greens ½ small tomato 2 Tbsp blue cheese dressing **Net Carbs: 3.7g; FV: 2.6g**	4–6 oz chicken 1 cup mixed greens ½ cup sliced bell pepper 2 Tbsp vinaigrette **Net Carbs: 2.7g; FV: 2.2g**
SNACK	1 medium tomato 2 oz pepper Jack cheese **Net Carbs: 5.3g; FV: 3.3g**	1 stalk celery 1 oz Cheddar cheese **Net Carbs: 1.4g; FV: 1**	½ cup sliced bell pepper 2 Tbsp ranch dressing **Net Carbs: 2.6g; FV: 1.9g**	1 small tomato 1 oz pepper Jack cheese **Net Carbs: 3.5g; FV: 2.5g**
DINNER	4–6 oz steak or hamburger 1 cup cauliflower florets 1 Tbsp butter 1 cup mixed greens 1 stalk celery 2 Tbsp vinaigrette **Net Carbs: 5.9g; FV: 5.5g**	4–6 oz canned tuna or fish filet 1 cup mixed greens ½ avocado 1½ oz mozzarella cheese 2 Tbsp creamy Italian dressing ½ cup green beans 1 Tbsp butter **Net Carbs: 7.1g; FV: 6.8g**	4–6 oz chicken ½ cup green beans 1 Tbsp butter 1 cup mixed greens ½ avocado 2 Tbsp creamy Italian dressing **Net Carbs: 5g; FV: 4.7g**	4–6 oz ham or pork chop 1 cup cauliflower florets 1 oz Cheddar cheese 2 cups mixed greens 2 Tbsp ranch dressing **Net Carbs: 7 g; FV: 5.9g**
	Total Net Carbs: 20.7g **Total Net Carbs from FV: 16.1g**	**Total Net Carbs: 18.7g** **Total Net Carbs from FV: 15.6g**	**Total Net Carbs: 19.5** **Total Net Carbs from FV: 15.7g**	**Total Net Carbs: 20.5g** **Total Net Carbs from FV: 16.9g**

Enjoy Atkins Endulge Treats for dessert if Net Carb consumption allows!

Friday	Saturday	Sunday
2 eggs	2 small tomatoes	2 eggs
½ avocado	2 oz bacon or sausage	½ avocado
1 oz pepper Jack cheese	1 oz Cheddar cheese	¼ cup chopped bell
⅛ cup salsa		pepper
		1 oz mozzarella cheese
Net Carbs: 4.6g; FV: 2.9g	**Net Carbs: 5.3g; FV: 4.9g**	**Net Carbs: 3.1g; FV: 2.4g**
1 small tomato	½ cup sliced bell pepper	2 stalks celery
2 Tbsp blue cheese	2 Tbsp ranch dressing	1 oz pepper Jack cheese
dressing		
Net Carbs: 3.2g; FV: 2.5g	**Net Carbs: 2.6g; FV: 1.9g**	**Net Carbs: 3g; FV: 2g**
4–6 oz canned tuna or	4–6 oz chicken	4–6 oz steak or
fish filet	1 cup cauliflower florets	hamburger
2 Tbsp mayonnaise or	1 Tbsp butter	1 cup mixed greens
Tartar Sauce	1 cup mixed greens	1 small tomato
1½ stalks celery	2 Tbsp vinaigrette	½ cup sliced bell pepper
3 cups mixed greens		½ avocado
½ avocado		2 Tbsp vinaigrette
2 Tbsp creamy Italian		
dressing		
Net Carbs: 7g; FV: 6.9g	**Net Carbs: 5g; FV: 4.5g**	**Net Carbs: 6.8g; FV: 6.5g**
½ cup sliced bell pepper	1 small tomato	1 small tomato
1 oz Cheddar cheese	2 oz mozzarella cheese	2 Tbsp blue cheese
		dressing
Net Carbs: 2.2g; FV: 1.9g	**Net Carbs: 2.5g; FV: 2.5g**	**Net Carbs: 3.2g; FV: 2.5g**
4–6 oz chicken	4–6 oz steak or hamburger	4–6 oz chicken
1 cup mixed greens	½ cup green beans	1 cup cauliflower florets
½ small tomato	1 Tbsp olive oil	1 Tbsp butter
2 Tbsp vinaigrette	1 cup mixed greens	1 cup mixed greens
	½ avocado	2 Tbsp creamy Italian
	2 Tbsp blue cheese	dressing
	dressing	
Net Carbs: 3g; FV: 2.5g	**Net Carbs: 5.4g; FV: 4.7g**	**Net Carbs: 4.8g; FV: 4.5g**
Total Net Carbs: 20g	**Total Net Carbs: 20.8g**	**Total Net Carbs: 20.9g**
Total Net Carbs from	**Total Net Carbs from**	**Total Net Carbs from**
FV: 16.7g	**FV: 18g**	**FV: 17.9g**

SHOPPING LIST FOR WEEK 2

WEEK 2

PROTEINS	DAIRY/CHEESE	VEGETABLES	SAUCES/CONDIMENTS	ATKINS PRODUCTS
Steak or Hamburgers	Butter	Hass Avocados	*Blue Cheese Dressing**	Atkins Bars
Chicken	Cheddar Cheese	*Green Beans*	*Salsa**	Atkins Shakes
Eggs	*Mozzarella Cheese*	Cauliflower florets	Creamy Italian Dressing*	Atkins Frozen Meals
Ham or Pork Chop	*Pepper Jack Cheese*	Celery	Mayonnaise or Tartar Sauce*	
Canned Tuna or Fish Fillet		Green or Red Bell Pepper	Ranch Dressing*	
Bacon or Sausages		Lettuce/ Mixed Greens	Vinaigrette*	
		Tomatoes	Extra Virgin Olive Oil	

* Select sauces and condiments without added sugar.

TIME TO EVALUATE YOUR PROGRESS

After two weeks on Atkins, you're practically an old hand! By now you're probably reaching your stride, losing inches and pounds. I'll bet you can now zip up your jeans all the way again! Once more, take your measurements and weigh yourself. Why are your measurements so important? Assuming that you're exercising, you may be gaining lean body mass and losing fat. Because muscle is denser than fat, the scale can be deceiving. How your clothes fit is another useful calculation. Even if your weight remains stable for a week or so, if your jeans zip up more easily, you're losing fat.

If all went well during your first week, in all likelihood you continued to lose weight this week. If so, you're definitely burning fat for energy. You've probably also banished cravings for unsuitable foods, are in control of your appetite, feel energized, and have said good-bye to any annoying symptoms if you ever had them. Keep up the good work. If you uncovered some glitches after the first week and have corrected them, the chances are good that your results have improved. It may have taken you a little longer to spark your fat-burning metabolism, but now you're on your way.

But what if you have made all of the recommended changes that could have been hindering weight loss in the first week but the pounds and inches refuse to budge? Sad to say, some people are highly resistant to weight loss, and you may simply be a slow starter. In addition to the issues discussed earlier, here are some possible reasons and suggestions for overcoming them:

- You're simply eating too much despite thinking your portions are appropriately sized. Review the guidelines on page 54 one more time and, rather than estimate, actually measure your portions and record them.
- You have high insulin levels. Insulin is the fat-storing hormone. It may simply take you longer to initiate fat burning by controlling carb intake.
- You have an underactive thyroid. If this has been a problem in the past or you suspect it may be now, discuss it with your physician.
- Your menstrual period is interfering with weight loss. Some women lose very slowly or not at all right before their period.
- Certain medications may interfere with weight loss. Review the list on page 45 and discuss alternatives with your health care provider.
- You're sedentary. Begin some form of exercise, such as walking or swimming, to see if that gets the pounds moving along with you.

BUDDY UP

Whether it's improving your tennis game or slimming down, it's definitely easier to achieve any goal if you're working with someone who has your back. That's what buddies are for. You'll be able to celebrate each other's victories as well as help each other regain equilibrium when forward momentum is lacking. A buddy also helps keep you in line, perhaps talking you off the ledge when a jelly doughnut beckons after a stressful day. In an ideal world, your buddy would be your gender and age, have about the same amount of weight to lose, and live down the street. That said, if you're both doing Atkins, your significant other might be a great buddy. A friend or relative in another town could do too, as could someone you meet in an Atkins chat room. With Skype, email, instant messaging, or tweets, you may never meet face-to-face with the person who's sharing your journey.

If you're having trouble sticking with the program, an Atkins buddy can be a huge help. If your problem is more one of perception than of compliance, accept that although you're losing more slowly than you'd hoped, you're heading in the right direction. For more on trouble-shooting in Phase 1 (Kick-Start), see the FAQs that follow.

FREQUENTLY ASKED QUESTIONS

Q. Can I eat more carbs one day if I cut back the next?
A. By maintaining a constant level of carb intake from day to day, you're more likely to keep your blood sugar on an even keel. But a range of 3 or 4 grams of Net Carbs from one day to the next should not create a problem as long as your average intake is consistent. If you do overindulge one day, simply return to your current level the next day.

Q. Why can't I do Atkins during the week and then take the weekend off?

A. Doing so will mean that you're consistently returning to a primarily blood sugar metabolism for two days. It then takes several days to re-ignite your fat-burning engine. Stopping and starting, known as "carb cycling," will lessen the likelihood that you'll lose weight or keep it off.

Q. Will drinking caffeinated beverages interfere with weight loss?
A. Caffeine itself doesn't slow weight loss. Drinking a few cups of coffee or tea each day actually produces numerous health benefits. However, have your beverages without sugar or honey. Noncaloric sweeteners are okay, but have no more than three packets a day. Also lighten these beverages with cream, half-and-half, or acceptable dairy substitutes, not milk.

Q. Can I consume beer, wine, or other alcohol in Phase 1?
A. No. However, once you transition to Phase 2, you can consume moderate amounts of most alcoholic beverages, assuming it doesn't interfere with weight loss, as we'll discuss in Chapter 5.

Q. If the object is to stay at 20 grams of Net Carbs a day, why can't I have Atkins bars and shakes or a slice of bread instead of all those vegetables?
A. You're not just tracking your carb intake; you're also aiming for a well-balanced meal plan full of vitamins and other nutrients provided by vegetables, along with fiber to help manage your hunger. One slice of bread might represent the balance of your daily carb intake in Phase 1, which would put your blood sugar back on the roller coaster.

Q. Why can't I drink tomato or orange juice with my breakfast?
A. The juicing process removes all or most of the fiber in fruit and vegetables, concentrating the sugar hit. You'll be able to introduce tomato juice in Phase 2. In Phase 3, oranges and other citrus fruits are acceptable.

Q. Why is cream allowed in Phase 1 but not milk?

A. Strange as it may seem, milk is higher in carbs than cream, thanks to the lactose (a form of sugar). In Phase 2 you can reintroduce small amounts of whole milk. Or dilute cream with some water, if you prefer.

Q. I'm experiencing cravings for sweets and other high-carb foods such as muffins, bread, and chips. How do I stay in control of my appetite?

A. Most likely your blood sugar levels have not yet stabilized, which usually occurs after the fifth day on Atkins. Once you're burning fat for energy, it acts as a natural appetite suppressant. Sometimes women have cravings right before their menstrual period. Or you may be going too long between meals or snacks, eating foods that contain hidden sugars or grains, or not consuming enough fat. When you experience cravings for high-carb foods, have an Atkins bar or shake, half a Hass avocado, some cheese, or some olives instead. Hunger and cravings can also be confused with thirst, so drink up.

In the next chapter, we'll tackle the all-important question of the right time to transition on to Phase 2 (Balancing) of the New Atkins Diet. For some of you it's likely to be after two weeks on the program. Or you may prefer to wait several weeks or even several months. It's your decision and many factors come into play, but I'll give you the pros and cons for each path so you can make the decision that's right for you.

Meanwhile, turn the page to meet Patricia O., who found some pounds returning after she'd kept them off for years. When she came to understand the changes she needed to make in order to stay on top of her weight and returned to her exercise regimen, the excess pounds beat a hasty retreat.

ATKINS PLUS EXERCISE ADDS UP
TO SUCCESS

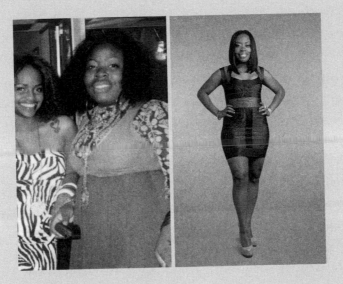

VITAL STATS

Daily Net Carb intake: 25 grams

Age: 25

Height: 5'5"

Before weight: 253 pounds

After weight: 152 pounds

Lost: 101 pounds

Nurse and aspiring physician Patricia O. lost weight six years ago on Atkins and kept it off while she was in nursing school. But after graduation she returned home to Houston, where juggling a demanding job while taking the college courses necessary to apply to medical school made it hard to stay on track. Finding time to exercise was almost impossible. It's not surprising that some of the lost weight returned. Working with the support of an Atkins nutritionist online, Patricia was able to banish the pounds again and begin a maintenance program she can stick with despite her hectic schedule. Here's her story.

I've dealt with weight issues all my life. I remember once being teased so badly at school for being heavy that I came home crying. When I told my father what the other kids had said to me, instead of comforting me, he agreed with them. My father's attitude didn't help my self-image. Once he and I were shopping and in front of a group of other girls, he said, "How come you can't look like them? Just look at yourself." It wasn't until later on in my life that I realized that was his way to motivate me to change my eating habits. Of course, losing weight was solely dependent on me to decide that I'd had enough of feeling bad about myself. Meanwhile, my mother would tell me to eat. I felt pulled in two directions.

I've always been an emotional eater, and I loved sweets, potatoes, mac and cheese, and anything white. By the time I graduated from high school, I weighed 204 pounds. Then, instead of the usual "freshman 15," I gained 50 pounds in my first year of nursing school, and my emotional state was terrible. Another nursing student introduced me to Atkins and told me what to eat and not eat. Doing Atkins put me more in control, so I was able to lose the excess weight and keep it off for three and a half years. I also began working out at the same time I started Atkins. In the process, I overcame my insecurities. One thing I knew for sure was that I never wanted to go back to that dark place where I was before!

That made it all the more upsetting when I started regaining lost weight. I was frustrated but knew I had to do something.

I had completed nursing school and was working full-time. I had decided to apply to medical school—I want to go into cardiology—but needed to take postgrad courses in physics and organic chemistry. There didn't seem to be enough hours in the day to handle work, school, and homework, plus establish a routine that allowed me to eat properly and exercise. I was doing Atkins during the week but bingeing on carbs on the weekend. Not surprisingly, I couldn't lose the 12 pounds I'd regained.

I now realize that I wasn't *really* doing Atkins—or I wasn't doing it correctly. I'd never read a book about why and how it works. And I didn't get it that Phase 1 was not the whole Atkins program. I thought I would just have to eat that way for the rest of my life to keep the weight off. After reading *The New Atkins for a New You* and getting a pep talk from an Atkins nutritionist, I was motivated to get on the right track. I started keeping a journal, added nuts to my meals, and slowly added other carb foods. I'm back to running 5 miles five times a week. I now know that staying active is key to maintaining my weight. Even thirty minutes a day makes a huge difference. My mood has lifted, and best of all, I've lost the weight I regained. And it wasn't even that hard! My next goal is to lose another 5 pounds. And now that I'm doing everything right, I know I will get there!

MAKE IT EASY

Always plan ahead. If you don't have the right food with you at all times, you may be tempted to eat whatever is handy. —*P.O.*

CHAPTER 5

WHAT'S NEXT? TRANSITION TO PHASE 2—OR NOT

After two weeks on Atkins, it's decision time. Assuming you've been following the program correctly and have lost weight over the last two weeks, you can choose to remain in Phase 1 (Kick-Start) or transition to Phase 2 (Balancing). Although you should spend a minimum of two weeks in the first phase to train your body to burn fat, initiating weight loss, there's no maximum limit. In the second phase, you'll get into the steady rhythm of weight loss that will carry you until you're 15 pounds from your goal weight. By then, you'll understand how your body reacts to certain foods and to gradual increases in carb intake. The decision about when you start to move up the Carb Ladder is a purely personal one.

Many people come to regard Phase 1 as a "security blanket," because for the first time in years they feel in control of what they put in their mouth. And their continuing positive results reinforce this inaction. However, at some point weight loss is bound to slow, even if you stay at 20 grams of Net Carbs a day. It can be a false security to feel that you cannot leave this phase. In the long run, it's essential to find out what you can eat while maintaining a healthy weight. Moving up the Carb Ladder enables you to do this. Learning a way to eat for a lifetime is the real objective of Atkins.

FACTORS TO CONSIDER

That said, you may remain in Phase 1 as long as you want, assuming you don't become bored with the food choices or get within 15 pounds of your goal weight. In fact, there's no health risk associated with staying in this phase indefinitely. (See "Carb Balancing—Steps to Weight Loss" on page 17 to visualize the two paths, known as Fast Track and Slow and Steady, described below.) The trick is not to get stuck there. Feel free to hang out in Phase 1 longer than two weeks if you have a lot of weight to lose. Weight loss typically slows after the initial dramatic drop that occurs when you switch to burning primarily fat for energy. But that natural slowdown is actually a good thing, as we'll discuss here. In addition to reducing the possibility of boredom, there's another reason why staying too long in Phase 1 can be a problem: you'll have no place to go if and when—and it's almost inevitable—you experience a weight-loss plateau. That's because you can't drop below 20 grams of Net Carbs a day without sacrificing foundation vegetables, which is not negotiable. (We'll discuss plateauing in Chapter 6.)

THE FAST TRACK

If you're motivated by quick weight loss and thrive on structure and a minimum of choices, you may choose to stay in Phase 1 beyond two weeks. To make this process easier, as well as set the stage for when you do decide to move on:

- Continue to consume 20 grams of Net Carbs a day beyond the first two weeks.

- Try adding nuts and seeds to your list of acceptable foods. Nuts are full of protein and healthy fats and are relatively low in Net Carbs, thanks to their high fiber content.
  - ▶ To make it easy, simply follow the meal plans on pages 62 and 64, swapping out 3 grams of Net Carbs from other foods, such as ½ cup of green beans, a smallish tomato, or 1½ cups mixed greens, for 3 grams of nuts or seeds, but without letting your intake of foundation veggies dip below 12 grams of Net Carbs. (You'll still have 5 grams for Atkins bars and shakes, sweeteners, dressings, or condiments.)
  - ▶ As a quick guide, 3 grams of Net Carbs of nuts or seeds translates to 30 almonds, 3 tablespoons macadamia nuts, 2 tablespoons peanut butter, 2 tablespoons pistachios, or 4 tablespoons shelled sunflower seeds; 24 walnut halves come in at 3.4 grams.
  - ▶ Portion out nuts and seeds in advance to avoid overeating. A couple of tablespoons of walnuts, almonds, pecans, or pumpkin seeds make a great snack. Or top a salad with sunflower seeds or chopped walnuts. You can also now have other nut and seed butters (stuff them into celery sticks) or coconut, almond, and other nut flours (available in the baking section or specialty foods aisle of the supermarket).
- Transition to Phase 2 (Balancing) no later than when you're within 15 pounds of your goal weight. At that point it's time to start transitioning to a permanent way of eating by introducing foods higher up the Carb Ladder.

Fast Track pros: Speedier weight loss, greater structure, and fewer choices, meaning fewer opportunities for temptation

Fast Track cons: Boredom; no options for moving past a plateau without reducing Net Carbs below the recommended level, which can be extremely frustrating and demotivating

SLOW AND STEADY

Alternatively, you may chose to lose the bulk of your weight in Phase 2 (Balancing), which Dr. Atkins dubbed Ongoing Weight Loss (OWL). If you're comfortable with a slower, steadier rate of weight loss, after two weeks (or a few more) start to climb the Carb Ladder (page 16). The gradual increase in Net Carb intake and reintroduction of new foods allows you to continue to shave off pounds and inches, maintain appetite control, and feel energetic. You'll also gradually come to understand which, if any, foods trigger cravings for more of the same and/or interfere with weight loss.

You may find that you're comfortable at a relatively low level of Net Carbs a day, perhaps 25 to 35 grams, which is not all that different from Kick-Start but does allow you to eat such delicious, nutritious food as nuts and seeds (see the meal plan for 25 grams of Net Carbs on page 118, for easy ways to add them) and then berries, melon, and cherries (see the meal plan for 30 grams of Net Carbs on page 134 for easy ways to add them). Next you'll move on to Greek yogurt and fresh cheeses (see page 115 for easy ways to add these "new" foods). Or you may find you can go considerably higher, say 50 or 60 grams of Net Carbs or even more, which will allow you to include legumes and some vegetable juices.

The balancing process enables you to find what works for you. Understanding your carb tolerance is the bridge from a weight-loss diet to a diet for life. This process can involve some fits and starts as you increase the variety of foods, but it's essential to understanding your unique metabolism. After all, wouldn't you rather lose a little more slowly and keep the weight off for good than lose rapidly by staying in Phase 1, reach your goal weight, and then regain those lost pounds because you never learned how to eat for the long run? Think of Atkins as a marathon rather than a sprint and you'll understand the rationale for losing the bulk of your weight in Phase 2 (Balancing).

Slow and Steady pros: More variety in what you can eat; more options for moving past a plateau because you can always return to a lower level of carb intake; easier segue to a sustainable way of eating

Slow and Steady cons: Slightly slower weight loss; having more food choices may be too tempting or confusing

WHICH PATH IS RIGHT FOR YOU?

Both these strategies will allow you to lose weight, but select the one that works best for you in the long run. By that I mean the option that will allow you to lose the weight—and then keep it off—while enjoying a satisfying way of eating. As you consider whether to leave the relative security of Induction to move on to Ongoing Weight Loss, ask yourself these questions.

- *Is routine important to you?* Are you in the habit of eating the same foods day after day? If your attitude is "Just tell me what to eat and I'm fine," you may actually find Atkins easier with a shorter list of acceptable foods, at least initially. Or do you get bored eating the same meals over and over again and delight in experimenting with new foods and new recipes?
- *Are you a tortoise or a hare?* Are you willing to take a bit longer to make the journey easier, or are you in a rush to get to your destination? Do you really miss eating berries or having a glass of wine, or can you put up with those limitations for the time being to get your weight under control sooner?
- *Do you miss certain foods?* If you might have a hard time moderating your intake of some foods beyond the first rungs of the Carb Ladder, you may want to hold off for now. Or if there's nothing there you can't live without for the time being, you may decide to wait. Or perhaps being able to have yogurt and berries for breakfast will make it easier to stay with Atkins.

- *What else is going on in your life?* If you're juggling work, a family, and school, for example, you may want to simplify things by staying with Phase 1 for the time being. Or perhaps for you, being able to eat a greater variety of foods is easier when other aspects of your life are stressful.

IT'S NOT JUST ABOUT WEIGHT

As you evaluate your experience in the first two weeks of Induction, look beyond just the changes in your weight and waistline. Those numbers are probably why you started Atkins, but consider other markers as well.

- If you have hypertension, has your blood pressure dropped? If your new way of eating is lowering it naturally and making you feel light-headed, be sure to talk to your health care provider—you likely need to reduce the dosage of your medication.
- If you are prediabetic or have type 2 diabetes, have your blood sugar levels improved? If so, it's crucial that you communicate that to your doctor in case it requires a change in your insulin or other medication dosage.
- Have your aches and pains diminished or vanished?
- Has your mood lifted?
- Are you in control of your appetite?

These factors are all part of the larger picture of how eliminating added sugar and other empty carbohydrates from your diet can improve your health and well-being. Even if your weight loss has been minimal, these indicators are clear evidence that Atkins is working for you.

TIME TO EXERCISE THE FITNESS OPTION?

Whether or not you decide to remain in Phase 1, after two weeks you may now want to add physical fitness to your weight-loss program. Regular physical activity is important for numerous reasons, among them:

- Maintaining cardiovascular health
- Keeping bones strong
- Lowering high blood pressure
- Boosting your metabolism
- Improving sleep quality
- Helping coordination and balance as you get older

If you already exercise regularly, whether walking briskly, taking Zumba or spinning classes, working out in a gym, or whatever, by all means continue to do so as long as your energy level remains high. It's not a good idea to simultaneously increase your current activity level or begin an intense fitness program as you start Atkins. However, once you get that burst of energy that usually occurs sometime within the first two weeks, ramp up your physical activity gradually.

What if you haven't been in the habit of exercising? I suggest you wait until you get comfortable with Atkins before starting or resuming a routine. After two weeks in Phase 1, that time may be right for you. If you've never been a "fitness freak" but want to test the waters, walking or swimming is the best way to begin. Start small, perhaps a quarter-mile walk before dinner or a few laps in the YMCA pool, and then increase your distances gradually. If you're extremely heavy, swimming is an excellent choice, because it causes minimal impact on your joints. Ditto for exercises you can do sitting in a chair.

Does that mean you *must* start some form of exercise after two weeks on Atkins whether or not you remain in Phase 1 or advance to Phase 2? No way. If your energy level is low or you simply aren't comfortable getting physical until you reduce your size, that's your choice. When and which kind of activity are personal decisions, but fitness is the natural partner to Atkins. So don't be surprised when I bring up exercise again in later chapters. Sooner or later you'll probably agree. As you'll hear from our success stories, most people found that as they slimmed down on Atkins, they became more interested in physical activity. Several of them, including Troy (page 146), have embraced competitive sports with a passion. Natalie (page 191) exercises "every single day, no matter what." Meanwhile, Joe (page 217), who has taught tae kwon do for years, no longer experiences excruciating pain after working out now that there is 200 pounds less of him!

Physical activity helps some people lose weight, but not everyone. However, it will reliably help you maintain your weight loss over the long term. The combination of following Atkins while engaging in regular physical exercise benefits body and mind by:

- Increasing your energy level
- Helping unlock your fat stores
- Inducing calmness
- Reducing stress
- Firming up flab
- Empowering you with a sense of mastery

Weight training or other strength-building exercise also helps build muscle, giving your body a more defined appearance. As a result, your clothes fit better. And the less fat and more muscle you have, the higher your metabolism, which means you burn more fat even when you're sitting or sleeping.

MOVING TO PHASE 2

If you've made the decision to take the Slow and Steady Track by step-ping up to Phase 2 (Balancing) sooner rather than later, you'll most likely spend the greatest amount of time in this phase as you continue to slim down. That's why it's designed to help you change habits as you gradually transition toward a permanent way of eating. You'll experi-ence greater freedom in this phase than in Phase 1 (Kick-Start). The trick is to exercise that freedom without undoing your initial results. The best way to handle that juggling act, what we call finding your personal carb balance, is to move slowly and deliberately up the Carb Ladder.

I can almost guarantee that if you rush to add back as many differ-ent foods as fast as you can, you'll stall your fat-burning engine. Worse, you could become discouraged and even give up on losing weight. Not to worry. I'm not going to let that happen to you. Nor need you retreat to the "safety net" of Phase 1. Here's how to succeed as you proceed up the Carb Ladder.

- Continue to consume a minimum of 12–15 daily grams of Net Carbs as foundation vegetables. Also continue to avoid foods with added sugar, have eight glasses of water or other accept-able fluids each day, and go no longer than three or four hours between meals or snacks, spreading out your carb intake across the day.
- Reintroduce food groups one by one, following the Carb Lad-der. Depending on your metabolism and weight-loss goal, this may be at weekly intervals, every couple of weeks, or even longer.
- Add back carb foods within each rung of the ladder one by one as well. For example, reintroduce walnuts but gauge their impact, if any, before reintroducing almonds.
- Increase your overall daily Net Carb intake in 5-gram increments

at weekly, biweekly, or even monthly intervals, whichever works best for you.

- Continue to track your daily Net Carb intake daily in your journal, also noting any new foods so that you can tell if they are stalling your progress.
- Continue to weigh and measure yourself weekly.

You may be reassured to see how similar Phase 1 (Kick-Start) is to Phase 2 (Balancing) initially. Again, proceeding slowly and deliberately will make it easy to transition from one phase to the next. In the following chapter, we'll get into greater detail on what to expect as you move forward, how to manage the food reintroduction process, and how to evaluate your responses to more carbs and a greater variety of foods.

CLIMBING THE CARB LADDER

In Phase 2, you'll start looking for your personal carb balance, increasing your Net Carb intake as you gradually reintroduce the foods on the five Phase 2 (Balancing) rungs of the Carb Ladder. (Since you can add nuts and seeds if you stay more than two weeks in Phase 1, they are not shown below.)

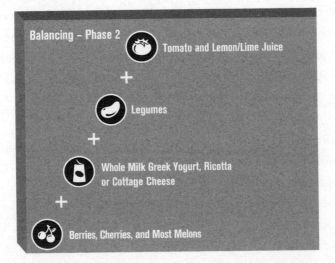

ACCEPTABLE PHASE 2 FOODS

Now, let's take a closer look at the acceptable Phase 2 foods incorporated in the Balancing process. Understand that you may not be able to reintroduce all of them in this phase. Nor may you be interested in eating all of them. The following lists are representative of each rung on the Carb Ladder. For a more complete list of options, complete with serving sizes and Net Carb gram counts, see the printed, online, or mobile app Atkins Carb Counter.

NUTS AND SEEDS

Peanuts, cashews, and soy "nuts" are not true nuts, but they can also be reintroduced in Phase 2. Do avoid chestnuts, which are very high in carbs, and salted nuts, which are notoriously difficult to eat in moderation. Also avoid products such as Nutella, which contains added sugars.

- Almonds
- Brazil nuts
- Cashews
- Coconut (fresh or grated and unsweetened)
- Macadamias
- Hazelnuts (also called filberts)

- Peanuts
- Pecans
- Pine nuts (also called piñons)
- Pistachios
- Pumpkin seeds (also called pepitas)
- Sesame seeds
- Soy "nuts"
- Sunflower seeds
- Walnuts

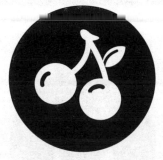

BERRIES, CHERRIES, AND MOST MELONS

The fruits suitable for OWL are lower in Net Carbs than most other fruits, because their fiber content is relatively high and fruit sugar content is relatively low. Still, have small portions and always accompany them with fat or protein. The following fruits can be fresh, frozen (as long as they're unsweetened), or canned in water or juice (but not syrup). You can also have 1-tablespoon portions of berry or cherry preserves that have no added sugar and are sweetened only with acceptable sweeteners.

- Blackberries, blueberries, boysenberries, fresh currants, gooseberries, loganberries, raspberries, and strawberries
- Cherries, sour or sweet

- Unsweetened cranberries and cranberry sauce made with acceptable sweeteners only
- Melon: cantaloupe, Crenshaw, and honeydew (but not watermelon)

MAKE IT EASY

Always have berries or other Phase 2 fruits with cheese, cream, Greek yogurt (acceptable in this phase), or nuts to temper their impact on your blood sugar. Or use them to garnish a salad—the oil in the dressing serves the same purpose. Melon with prosciutto is a classic fruit-and-protein combo.

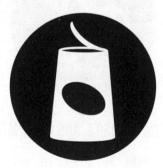

MORE DAIRY OPTIONS

In addition to Phase 1 cheeses (page 36) and additional dairy products and dairy substitutes (page 37), your options now expand. Always select whole-milk or full-fat dairy products, including yogurt. Low-fat dairy products are higher in carbs.

- Cottage cheese (not low-fat), creamed or curd style
- Ricotta cheese, whole-milk
- Yogurt or Greek yogurt, whole-milk, plain, unsweetened

- Whole milk, fresh (limit to 4 tablespoons) or evaporated (limit to 2 tablespoons)

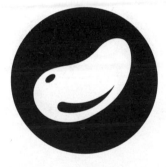

LEGUMES

Most legumes are sold dried, although a few, such as green soybeans (edamame) and baby lima beans, are usually sold fresh or frozen. (Green and wax beans are foundation vegetables, as are snow peas, meaning they are acceptable in Phase 1.) Avoid products such as baked beans made with added sugar. Hummus is a fine choice, but watch out for bean dips made with sugar or starches. You may choose to wait to reintroduce legumes until you move to Phase 3.

- Black beans (also called turtle beans)
- Black-eyed peas

- Chickpeas (also called garbanzo beans)
- Edamame
- Fava beans
- Great northern beans
- Hummus
- Kidney beans
- Lima beans
- Peas, split
- Pinto beans
- Soybeans

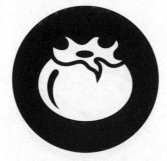

TOMATO AND LEMON/LIME JUICE

In Phase 1 you could have 2 tablespoons lemon or lime juice; now you can have:

- ¼ cup lemon or lime juice
- ½ cup tomato juice or tomato juice cocktail

All other fruit and vegetable juices remain off-limits.

FOOLPROOF ADVICE TO STAY IN CONTROL

Understand that as you move through the phases and up the Carb Ladder, your objective is not to increase the *amount* of food you eat, but instead to introduce greater variety. In many cases this means that you'll be making substitutions rather than additions. To stay in control of your appetite as you reintroduce carb foods:

- Put aside certain foods in the morning, such as 20 pecan or walnut halves or 4 large strawberries, to incorporate into your accustomed Induction meals.
- Add pepitas or sunflower seeds to salads rather than eating them out of hand.
- Swap out aged cheeses for fresh cheeses.
- Treat berries and melon as garnishes—perhaps a couple of strawberries atop a salad or a slice of melon wrapped in ham as part of your lunch.
- Top berries with Greek yogurt instead of whipped cream.
- Stir a couple of tablespoons of plain Greek yogurt into steamed spinach.
- Combine yogurt with mayo when making egg or tuna salad.
- Stuff celery sticks with hummus instead of cream cheese.
- Have a small glass of tomato juice in lieu of sliced tomatoes with your breakfast eggs.
- Instead of radishes or bell pepper slices, pair edamame with a piece of cheese as a snack.

ATKINS FOR VEGETARIANS

If you're a vegetarian, I recommend that you start Atkins in Phase 2 (Balancing), at 25–30 grams of Net Carbs a day so that you can get sufficient protein. Most vegetarian sources of protein also contain carbs, unlike most animal products. Read the chapters on Induction, but include nuts and seeds from the start. The following protein products are acceptable, but check the Nutrition Facts panel and the Atkins Carb Counter for Net Carb counts and serving sizes. Veggie burgers, for example, can vary dramatically in carb count, depending upon ingredients.

- Quorn cutlets, burgers, roast (unbreaded only)
- Tofu: firm, silken, or soft (not marinated)
- Tofu bacon, Canadian bacon, hot dogs, or sausage
- Tempeh (without grains)
- Seitan
- Shirataki soy noodles
- Veggie burgers, crumbles, or meatballs

PHASE 2 LOW-CARB PRODUCTS

Although not part of the Carb Ladder, certain low-carb products can be introduced in this phase, including the Atkins All Purpose Baking Mix and any remaining Atkins shakes or bars with Net Carb counts higher than 3 grams. You may also be able to have, in moderation, products such as low-carb bread, tortillas, wraps, or chips with no more than 6 grams of Net Carbs per serving. Atkins cannot vouch for the carb counts or ingredients in other companies' products, so study the Nutrition Facts panel and ingredient list carefully to assess the Net Carb count and find any added sugar or other unacceptable ingredients. If any of these foods provoke cravings, stop eating them for the time being. For more detail, see the Atkins Carb Counter.

WEEK-AT-A-GLANCE MEAL PLAN FOR WEEK 1 OF PHASE 2

As in Phase 1, you'll spread your carb intake out across the day to keep your blood sugar on an even keel. You'll continue to enjoy the protein, foundation vegetables, and acceptable Phase 1 dairy products you've been eating, but you'll add nuts and/or seeds. To make this transition easy, we've modified the Week 1 Phase 1 meal plan to show you how to include about 5 grams of Net Carbs of nuts or seeds each day (shown in boldface italic type). Your daily intake should range from 23–27 grams of Net Carbs, averaging out to 25. As with earlier meal plans, feel free to modify this one to suit your preferences, substituting your own recipes or those in the section starting on page 245.

Atkins Phase 2 (Balancing) Meal Plan at 25g NC/day

	Monday	Tuesday	Wednesday	Thursday

BREAKFAST	2 eggs
	¼ cup chopped onion
	1 tsp olive oil
	1 oz Cheddar cheese
	
	Net Carbs: 4.1g; FV: 3.1g
		Atkins Advantage Peanut
		  Butter Granola Bar
		25 almonds
		
		Net Carbs: 5.8g; FV: 0g
			Atkins Frozen
			  Farmhouse-Style
			  Sausage Scramble
			
			Net Carbs: 5g; FV: 1g
				4 oz steak or hamburger
				1 tsp olive oil
				½ cup chopped bell
				  pepper
				¼ cup chopped onion
				1 oz Cheddar cheese
				Net Carbs: 5.6g; FV: 5.3g

SNACK	Atkins Advantage Vanilla
	  Shake
	25 almonds
	Net Carbs: 3.8g; FV: 0g
		1 small tomato
		1 oz Monterey Jack
		  cheese
		Net Carbs: 2.6g; FV: 2.5g
			¾ cup sliced bell pepper
			2 Tbsp ranch dressing
			10 walnut halves
			Net Carbs: 4.9g; FV: 2.8g
				Atkins Advantage Milk
				  Chocolate Delight Shake
				15 walnut halves
				Net Carbs: 4.1g; FV: 0g

LUNCH	Atkins Frozen Crustless
	  Chicken Pot Pie
	
	Net Carbs: 5g; FV: 4g
		4–6 oz chicken
		1 small tomato
		1 cup mixed greens
		½ avocado
		2 Tbsp ranch dressing
		20 almonds
		
		Net Carbs: 8g; FV: 5.1g
			Atkins Frozen Beef
			  Merlot
			
			Net Carbs: 6g; FV: 4g
				4–6 oz ham or
				  pork chop
				1 cup baby spinach
				½ avocado
				1 Tbsp ranch dressing
				
				Net Carbs: 3.5g; FV: 2.8g

SNACK	Atkins Advantage Coconut
	  Almond Delight Bar
	20 almonds
	Net Carbs: 5.3g; FV: 0g
		1 stalk celery
		1 oz Cheddar cheese
		
		Net Carbs: 1.4g; FV: 1g
			Atkins Advantage
			  Café Caramel Shake
			25 almonds
			Net Carbs: 4.8g; FV: 0g
				1 small tomato
				2 Tbsp vinaigrette
				25 almonds
				Net Carbs: 5.7g; FV: 2.5g

DINNER	4–6 oz canned tuna or
	  fish filet
	2 cups mixed greens
	½ avocado
	2 Tbsp vinaigrette
	1 cup broccoli florets
	
	Net Carbs: 5.9g; FV: 5.6g
		Atkins Frozen Meatloaf
		  with Portobello
		  Mushroom Gravy
		
		Net Carbs: 7g; FV: 4g
			4–6 oz chicken
			1 cup broccoli florets
			1 Tbsp olive oil
			2 cups mixed greens
			2 Tbsp creamy Italian
			  dressing
			
			Net Carbs: 4.5g; FV: 4.3g
				Atkins Frozen Chicken and
				  Broccoli Alfredo
				
				Net Carbs: 5g; FV: 5g

	Total Net Carbs: 24.1g
	Total Net Carbs from
	  FV: 12.7g
		Total Net Carbs: 24.8g
		Total Net Carbs from
		  FV: 12.6g
			Total Net Carbs: 25.2g
			Total Net Carbs from
			  FV: 12.1g
				Total Net Carbs: 23.9g
				Total Net Carbs from
				  FV: 15.6g

Enjoy Atkins Endulge Treats for dessert if Net Carb consumption allows!

Friday	Saturday	Sunday

1 cup baby spinach
1 small tomato
½ avocado
1 oz Monterey Jack
  cheese
25 almonds
Net Carbs: 8.2g; FV: 5.3g
	Atkins Frozen Tex-Mex
	  Scramble
	
	Net Carbs: 5g; FV: 3g
		2 eggs
		2 cups baby spinach
		1 Tbsp olive oil
		½ bell pepper
		1 oz Monterey Jack
		  cheese
		Net Carbs: 6.2g; FV: 5.3g

2 oz Cheddar cheese 1 small tomato 2 Tbsp vinaigrette **Net Carbs: 3.6g; FV: 2.5g**	Atkins Advantage Caramel Chocolate Nut Roll Bar *15 walnut halves* **Net Carbs: 5.1g; FV: 0g**	1 stalk celery 1 oz Cheddar cheese **Net Carbs: 1.4g; FV: 1g**

Atkins Frozen Roast
  Turkey Tenders
  with Herb Pan Gravy
 	
Net Carbs: 6g; FV: 4g
	4–6 oz canned tuna or
	  fish filet
	2 Tbsp mayonnaise or
	  tartar sauce
	1 stalk celery
	¼ cup chopped bell
	  pepper
	1 small tomato
	Net Carbs: 5g; FV: 5g
		Atkins Advantage
		  Chocolate Peanut
		  Butter Bar
		20 walnut halves
		
		Net Carbs: 4.8g; FV: 0g

Atkins Advantage Caramel
  Chocolate Peanut
  Nougat Bar
Net Carbs: 3g; FV: 0g
	Atkins Advantage Vanilla
	  Shake
	25 almonds
	Net Carbs: 3.8g; FV: 0g
		½ cup chopped bell
		  pepper
		2 Tbsp ranch dressing
		Net Carbs: 2.9g; FV: 2.2g

4–6 oz ham or
  pork chop
1 cup broccoli
1 cup mixed greens
2 Tbsp creamy Italian
  dressing
10 walnut halves
Net Carbs: 4.6g; FV: 2.9g
	4 oz steak or hamburger
	1 small tomato
	½ avocado
	½ small onion, sliced
	
	Net Carbs: 6.4g; FV: 6.4g
		Atkins Frozen Crustless
		  Chicken Pot Pie
		25 almonds
		
		Net Carbs: 7.8g; FV: 4g

Total Net Carbs: 25.4g **Total Net Carbs from** **FV: 14.7g**	**Total Net Carbs: 25.3g** **Total Net Carbs from** **FV: 14.4g**	**Total Net Carbs: 23.1g** **Total Net Carbs from** **FV: 12.5g**

To update your shopping list, simply add the two items in boldface to your Week 1 shopping list. Also add any foods resulting from your modifications to the meal plan for this week.

PHASE 2 (BALANCING) WEEK 1

PROTEINS	DAIRY/CHEESE	VEGETABLES	CONDIMENTS/NUTS	ATKINS PRODUCTS
Steak or Hamburgers	Butter	Hass Avocados	Creamy Italian Dressing*	Atkins Bars
Chicken	Cheddar Cheese	Baby Spinach	Mayonnaise* or Tartar Sauce*	Atkins Shakes
Eggs	Monterey Jack Cheese	Broccoli Florets	Ranch Dressing*	Atkins Frozen Meals
Ham or Pork Chops		Celery	Vinaigrette*	
Canned Tuna or Fish Filets		Lettuce/ Mixed Greens	Extra Virgin Olive Oil	
Bacon		Onions	*Almonds*	
Sausages		Green or Red Bell Peppers	*Walnuts*	
		Tomatoes		

* Select sauces and condiments without added sugar.

TO DRINK OR NOT TO DRINK? THAT IS THE QUESTION

Alcoholic beverages are permissible in Phase 2 (Balancing). But your body burns alcohol, just as it does carbohydrate and fat. In fact, it burns alcohol before fat and after blood sugar (from carbs). So drinking wine, beer, or spirits delays fat burning. Although white and brown spirits (whiskey, rum, gin, vodka, etc.) contain no carbs, a 3½-ounce serving of white, red, or dry dessert wine contains 1, 2, or 4 grams of carbs, respectively. An ounce of spirits or a glass of wine is not going to have a big impact on your daily carb tally, but beer is another story. A 12-ounce can or bottle of most beer contains upward of 13 grams of carbs. Low-carb or "lite" beer cuts that to roughly 2.5 or 5.6 grams, respectively. Avoid wine coolers and conventional mixers, which are full of sugar. Fortunately, there are quite a few sugar-free mixers available.

So should you drink once you reach OWL? That depends.

- Can you stop at one drink (for women) or two drinks (for men)?
- Are you willing to drink spirits neat, with club soda or water, or with a sugar-free mixer?
- Can you moderate your intake of snacks such as salted peanuts or any other food when imbibing?

If the answer to any of these questions is no, you're probably better off waiting until you're closer to your goal weight to reintroduce alcohol.

CHEERS, SUGAR-FREE!

Most cocktails present liquid trouble. A 3½-ounce margarita, for example, racks up almost 14 grams of Net Carbs, and a piña colada more than 22 grams. But here's the good news. The following companies make sugar-free mixers for various drinks. Not every company offers every option, but you'll be able to find mixers for a bloody Mary, daiquiri, mai tai, margarita, cranberry or sour apple martini, mojito, mudslide, piña colada, and sweet and sour:

- Baja Bob's sugar-free cocktail mixers; bajabob.com
- Scales Cocktails; scalescocktails.com
- Lt. Blender's sugar-free cocktail mixers; ltblender.com
- Master of Mixes Lite Mixes; masterofmixes.com/lite

THE SCOOP ON SUGAR: PRIME OFFENDERS

Added sugars are found in countless common foods. Here's the (not so) skinny on a few that you may have been eating and drinking before you began Atkins, starting with those in which you wouldn't expect to find sugar and ending with those in which it's a key ingredient. Prepare to be astounded!

FOOD	SERVING	SUGAR CONTENT
Skippy Peanut Butter	2 tablespoons	3 grams
Kikkoman Seasoned Rice Vinegar	1 tablespoon	4 grams
Burger King Sweet and Sour Dipping Sauce	1 packet	10 grams
Nature Valley Trail Mix Chewy Granola Bar	1 bar	12 grams
Bush's Original Baked Beans	½ cup	12 grams
Campbell's Condensed Tomato Soup	½ cup	12 grams
Glacéau Vitamin Water	20 ounces	31 grams
Health Valley Apple Cobbler Cereal Bar	1 bar	16 grams
KFC Sweet & Spicy Wings	5.6 ounces	15 grams
Kikkoman Hoisin Sauce	2 tablespoons	17 grams
Libby's Easy Pumpkin Pie Mix	⅓ cup	17 grams
Snapple Iced Tea	8 ounces	18 grams
McDonald's Fruit 'N Yogurt Parfait	5.2 ounces	23 grams
Dannon Low-Fat Coffee Yogurt	6 ounces	26 grams
Ocean Spray Cranberry Juice	8 ounces	30 grams
Aunt Jemima Original Pancake Syrup	¼ cup	32 grams

FREQUENTLY ASKED QUESTIONS

Q. How long do I need to continue with salty broth or another salt source?

A. As long as you're no longer having symptoms of dehydration or electrolyte imbalance such as fatigue, dizziness upon standing, leg cramps, or constipation, you can stop, regardless of whether you stay in Phase 1 or transition to Phase 2. Continue to salt your food normally and drink plenty of fluids. Feel free to continue with the broth if you find it filling and soothing.

Q. I've had trouble transitioning from weight loss to weight maintenance in the past. How can I keep the pounds off this time?
A. If you previously lost all your excess weight in Phase 1 before trying to maintain your new weight, I strongly suggest you follow the Slow and Steady path this time. In Chapter 8, you'll find techniques to help you stay in control over the long term.

Q. If I miss berries more than nuts and seeds, can I add them back first?
A. As long as you can control your portions and proceed with caution, you can reorder the introduction of Phase 2 (Balancing) acceptable foods on the Carb Ladder. However, nuts and seeds are full of protein and fat, making them more satiating than berries, although both are relatively low in carbs.

Q. If I'm extremely overweight, is it safe to exercise?
A. Yes, in general, but consult with your physician first. Once you have the go-ahead, your best bets are activities that don't stress your joints, such as chair exercises, swimming, pedaling a reclining stationary bike, and water exercises. Walking and bike riding are also good choices.

Q. How can I determine the carb count of a restaurant meal?
A. Most casual dining and fast-food chains offer nutritional data online, so you can decide ahead of time what to order. (You may have to subtract fiber from total carbs to get Net Carbs.) Some apps allow you to subtract or add certain items such as a roll, mustard, or tomato on a burger, for example, or see the impact of grilled chicken with and

without fries. Certain states and municipalities also require that nutritional data be provided or posted. Nonetheless, you're often on your own, which is where the Atkins mobile app and Atkins Carb Counter come to the rescue.

In the next chapter, we'll discuss how to gradually move up the Carb Ladder, reintroducing more variety and more grams of Net Carbs back into your meals as you continue to slim down. This is all part of finding your personal carb balance. We'll also probe how to troubleshoot a weight-loss plateau and other issues. But before that, let me introduce you to Heather H., whose embarrassment over her size had made her a virtual hermit. Before embarking on Atkins, she did her homework to make sure she knew how to do it right. And she has, as her impressive results make clear.

PREPARATION IS THE SECRET TO SUCCESS

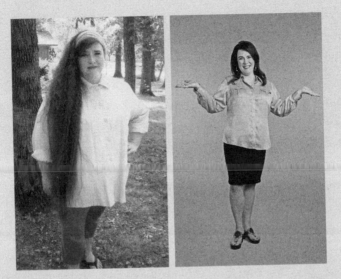

VITAL STATS

Daily Net Carb intake: 20 grams

Age: 43

Height: 5'5½"

Before weight: 330 pounds

After weight: 195 pounds

Lost: 135 pounds

Heather H. had spent her thirties hiding from life, too embarrassed to go out in public. During that time the Mountain Home, Arkansas, resident had developed type 2 diabetes, along with diabetic kidney disease, high cholesterol, and severe sleep apnea. Although Heather had tried other diets, including Atkins, without success, the idea of facing her forties in the same sorry shape was unacceptable. She was ready to enjoy life, and she knew Atkins was the key that would open that door. Heather relates her inspiring tale.

I had always been a big girl, but I was in a terrible marriage and really let myself go. My endocrinologist said that although my kidney disease was in an early stage, if I didn't get in shape I could lose one or more limbs. The only thing that was going well was my work. I work at home developing software for public education. I had done Atkins in 2003 and lost 60 pounds, but after having a miscarriage, I regained the weight.

What did I eat? The better question is what didn't I eat. I'd have potatoes, bread, sweets, cookies, and all the other things that were wrong for my metabolism. I was never a moody eater and I'd eat regularly, but my meals were two or three times as large as a normal meal.

When I was ready to lose the weight once and for all, I took my time. I spent two months reading *The New Atkins for a New You*, finding low-carb recipes, and planning menus. I also started preparing for a total life change. I knew that once I started I would remain on Atkins forever. Potatoes, pasta, and pastries are just not an option for my body. I also started walking for thirty to forty minutes every day around the neighborhood.

I began Atkins in May 2011, the day after my forty-first birthday. My family was wonderfully supportive. Within six months I'd lost 95 pounds, my blood sugar levels were excellent, my cholesterol had improved, and I am no longer classified as having diabetic kidney disease. I'm also able to sleep again without the aid of the CPAP (continuous positive airway pressure) mask. The weight comes off more slowly now, but I've lost 135 pounds and am working toward my goal weight of 175 pounds.

I'm totally into Atkins, but I'm not really into cooking. And I'm not really a breakfast person, so I usually have an Atkins bar—my favorites are the Peanut Butter Fudge and the brownies—or a shake instead. I always read labels, and believe me, sugar is everywhere. I have the Atkins Carb Counter app on my smartphone, which really helps me, especially when I'm eating at a new place. I also have menus from all over for takeout. As I said, I like to be prepared!

How much I weigh is not as much of an issue to me as my health and how I feel. Still, I've gone from wearing size 6X jeans to size 12. Yay! It feels so nice to be able to breathe, to tie my shoelaces, to get into a car and not have to push the seat all the way back to fit in. Even little things like riding a bike and being able to sit comfortably in a movie theater or restaurant are simply amazing! I've regained my confidence and am no longer ashamed to be seen in public.

Losing weight helped me make the decision to divorce my husband. Dating again is strange but fun. My daughter is so proud of me, and I'm proud to be a role model for her. For the first time in twelve years I really want to get out and do things. I feel great and I want to see the world—and the world to see me!

MAKE IT EASY

Be sure there's always plenty of food in the house by cooking up a big batch, so when you get hungry, you aren't tempted to eat the wrong thing. Peanuts are my favorite snack. Just be sure to portion them out in 1-ounce bags. —H.H.

CHAPTER 6

BEGIN TO FIND YOUR PERSONAL CARB BALANCE

I'll bet you're looking forward to savoring strawberries, blueberries, melon, cottage cheese, yogurt, and more, along with the nuts and seeds you've probably already reintroduced. If you've chosen to take the Slow and Steady path by starting to climb the Carb Ladder, you'll begin to explore these and other foods that will add delicious variety to your meals. (If you've chosen the Fast Track, see "Remaining in Phase 1—for Now," page 130.) Patience is essential for an easy transition from Phase 1 (Kick-Start) to Phase 2 (Balancing).

Instead of adding these foods all at once, start with the berries and other acceptable fruits listed on page 111, introducing them one by one. Wait a couple of days at the very least after you reintroduce blueberries, for example, before trying strawberries or cantaloupe, to gauge your response. If one fruit doesn't cause cravings or stimulate your appetite for more, try another. Then, and only then, move on to the dairy products listed on page 112, at the same time increasing your daily Net Carb intake by 5 grams. By slowly exploring greater flexibility and freedom of choice as you move up the Carb Ladder, you can ease from one phase to the next while continuing to experience the empowering sense of control to which you've become accustomed.

You'll use this latitude to begin the process of finding your personal carb balance, the amount and variety of carb foods you can consume while continuing to lose weight, feel great, and remain in control of your appetite. If you're on the Slow and Steady path, you're likely to spend a significant amount of time and lose most of your excess weight in Phase 2. Depending upon how sensitive you are to carbs and how much weight you want to lose, this could take anywhere from several weeks to a number of months. But regardless of the amount of time it takes, follow the rungs of the Carb Ladder and the suggestions below to ease the process.

WHAT TO EXPECT IN PHASE 2

Initially Phase 2 (Balancing) of the New Atkins is very similar to Phase 1 (Kick-Start). You take the first baby step as you increase to 25 daily grams of Net Carbs. As long as you anticipate certain situations, you'll retain that sense of control over your appetite and intake, although you may have to make some midcourse corrections. You'll likely experience several things in this phase.

- *The pace of your weight loss may slow.* Unless you have lots of weight to shed, the rapid weight loss that you may have experienced in the initial phase usually slows down. This may not happen immediately, but when it eventually does, be prepared, understand that it's perfectly normal, and adjust your expectations accordingly. After all, as you slim down, each banished pound represents a greater percentage of your remaining weight. And weight is only one measure of your success. Equally important are your energy level and mood.

- *Your hunger level may increase.* As you add more carbs and reintroduce certain foods you may find yourself hungrier than you were in Induction. This makes it all the more important that you not go too long between meals and snacks and continue to eat the recommended amounts of protein and fat.
- *Cravings may return.* After thinking you were permanently rid of the cravings that almost miraculously disappeared in your weeks in Induction, you may find that it's hard to stop eating certain foods or they make you crave other carb foods. We'll discuss how to deal with cravings below.
- *You may experience weight-loss plateaus.* This can happen at any time but is increasingly likely the longer you spend losing weight. Your body has its own internal logic, as you'll learn in "A Plateau Calls for Patience," page 140.

REMAINING IN PHASE 1—FOR NOW

If you've decided to stay at 20 grams of Net Carbs for the time being but have added back nuts and seeds, read this chapter to learn what to expect when the time comes to transition to Phase 2. Again, you should do so *no later* than when you're 15 pounds from your goal weight. On page 140, I'll address the issue of weight-loss plateaus while you're still in Phase 1. Remember, you can move to Phase 2 at any time if you desire more variety in your carb choices.

EVALUATE YOUR FIRST WEEK IN PHASE 2

If you followed the guidelines in the previous chapter (page 108) to the letter, you probably found your first week smooth sailing. However, if you overdid things—perhaps overindulging in peanuts, for example— you may need to rein in your enthusiasm. Also, if you have a very low tolerance for carbs, even the slight increase to 25 daily grams of Net Carbs might have slowed down weight loss. Let's try to tease out whether all is well or you need to make a minor adjustment. Start out with your usual weekly weigh-in and measurements. Then answer these questions.

- *Did you lose any weight?* If so, and if you can say with certainty that you're doing Phase 2 (Balancing) properly, relax. If the number on the scale didn't represent as great a loss as the week before, understand that you cannot expect to lose the same amount of weight week after week, particularly once you leave the initial phase of Atkins.
- *Did you lose inches?* Once again, inches often disappear before pounds and are a good indicator that you're moving in the right direction.
- *Did you lose neither weight nor inches?* If so, review the guidelines on page 108 to be sure that you're doing everything correctly and not overdoing serving sizes.
- *Are you experiencing cravings?* If any food causes cravings, stop eating it for several days before trying to reintroduce it. If you find it hard to stop with a few almonds, or that an hour after you eat a small portion of blueberries you're just dying for more, you need to act—fast. Note these events in your journal, along with whether (and how) you were able to control the cravings. Perhaps you ate those berries "naked" the first time before realizing you're better off serving them with whipped cream or nuts. Or you dug into a supersized container of almonds instead of putting 1 ounce into a small resealable bag.
- *Are you hungrier than you were in Induction?* Stay alert to hunger signals; if and when they hit, have a low-carb snack. Or eat your next meal a little earlier than you might have otherwise.

MOVING TO WEEK 2 OF PHASE 2

Your results in the first week will determine your actions as you move into Week 2. If you lost pounds and inches and weren't plagued anew with cravings and undue hunger, you may feel comfortable moving up to 30 grams of daily Net Carbs after just a week. If you wish, you can also move up one rung on the Carb Ladder (see page 109) and begin eating berries, cherries, and most kinds of melon. (See the meal plan on page 134.) However, if your weight loss slowed and you found it more difficult to stay in control, you're better off remaining at 25 grams of Net Carbs without going up another rung on the Carb Ladder. Instead, for variety, you could play with introducing other nuts and/or seeds. This will give your system time to adapt to these foods and the slightly higher carb intake of OWL.

Don't regard a slowdown in your weekly weight loss as a defeat, and don't rush back to the security of Phase 1 (Kick-Start). Depending upon the efficiency of your fat-burning engine, you may be able to climb the Carb Ladder quickly and increase your daily Net Carb intake every week or so, or you may proceed much more slowly. Small moves enable you to remain in control. Tailor your journey based on your weekly weight and inch loss and your response to foods on different steps of the ladder.

WEEK-AT-A-GLANCE MEAL PLAN AT 30 GRAMS OF NET CARBS

The meal plan on page 134 represents the second step up the Carb Ladder (see page 109). You'll continue to enjoy the Phase 1 (Kick-Start) foods, as well as the nuts and/or seeds you've recently added. The only difference is that you'll add about 5 grams of Net Carbs from the berries and other low-carb fruits listed on page 111.

To make this transition easy, we've again modified the original meal plan to show how to include the berries, cherries, and melon rung of the Carb Ladder. See the simple suggestions indicated in boldface italics in the meal plan on page 118 for how to add back these foods. (They are also in boldface italic type on the shopping list below.) Additions are small and incremental, ensuring that changes take place slowly, which moderates any impact on your blood sugar level. Feel free to substitute other Phase 2 fruits for the items listed, using the Atkins Carb Counter to check their carb counts.

PHASE 2 (BALANCING), WEEK 1

PROTEINS	DAIRY/CHEESE	VEGETABLES	CONDIMENTS/NUTS	ATKINS PRODUCTS/FRUIT
Steak or Hamburgers	Butter	Hass Avocados	Creamy Italian Dressing*	Atkins Bars
Chicken	Cheddar Cheese	Baby Spinach	Mayonnaise* or Tartar Sauce*	Atkins Shakes
Eggs	Monterey Jack Cheese	Broccoli Florets	Ranch Dressing*	Atkins Frozen Meals
Ham or Pork Chops		Celery	Vinaigrette*	*Strawberries*
Canned Tuna or Fish Filets		Lettuce/ Mixed Greens	Extra Virgin Olive Oil	*Cantaloupe*
Bacon or Sausages		Onions	Almonds	*Raspberries*
		Green or Red Bell Peppers	Walnuts	
		Tomatoes		

* Select sauces and condiments without added sugar.

Atkins Phase 2 (Balancing) Meal Plan at 30g NC/day

	Monday	Tuesday	Wednesday	Thursday

BREAKFAST	2 eggs
	¼ cup chopped onion
	1 tsp olive oil
	1 oz Cheddar cheese
	
	Net Carbs: 4.1g; FV: 3.1g
		Atkins Advantage Peanut
		  Butter Granola Bar
		25 almonds
		5 large strawberries
		
		Net Carbs: 11g; FV: 0g
			Atkins Frozen
			  Farmhouse-Style
			  Sausage Scramble
			⅓ *cup cantaloupe cubes*
			
			Net Carbs: 8.9g; FV: 1g
				4 oz steak or hamburger
				1 tsp olive oil
				½ cup chopped bell
				  pepper
				¼ cup chopped onion
				1 oz Cheddar cheese
				Net Carbs: 5.6g; FV: 5.3g

SNACK	Atkins Advantage
	  Vanilla Shake
	25 almonds
	5 large strawberries
	Net Carbs: 9g; FV: 0g
		1 small tomato
		1 oz Monterey Jack
		  cheese
		
		Net Carbs: 2.6g; FV: 2.5g
			¾ cup sliced bell pepper
			2 Tbsp ranch dressing*
			10 walnut halves
			
			Net Carbs: 4.9g; FV: 2.8g
				Atkins Advantage Milk
				  Chocolate Delight Shake
				15 walnut halves
				
				Net Carbs: 4.1g; FV: 0g

LUNCH	Atkins Frozen Crustless
	  Chicken Pot Pie
	
	Net Carbs: 5g; FV: 4g
		4–6 oz chicken
		1 small tomato
		1 cup mixed greens
		½ avocado
		2 Tbsp ranch dressing
		20 almonds
		
		Net Carbs: 8g; FV: 5.1g
			Atkins Frozen Beef
			  Merlot
			
			Net Carbs: 6g; FV: 4g
				4–6 oz ham or
				  pork chop
				1 cup baby spinach
				½ avocado
				1 Tbsp ranch dressing
				
				Net Carbs: 3.5g; FV: 2.8g

SNACK	Atkins Advantage Coconut
	  Almond Delight Bar
	20 almonds
	Net Carbs: 5.3g; FV: 0g
		1 stalk celery
		1 oz Cheddar cheese
		
		Net Carbs: 1.4g; FV: 1g
			Atkins Advantage
			  Café Caramel Shake
			25 almonds
			Net Carbs: 4.8g; FV: 0g
				1 small tomato
				2 Tbsp vinaigrette
				25 almonds
				Net Carbs: 5.7g; FV: 2.5g

DINNER	4–6 oz canned tuna or
	  fish filet
	2 cups mixed greens
	½ avocado
	2 Tbsp vinaigrette
	1 cup broccoli florets
	
	Net Carbs: 5.9g; FV: 5.6g
		Atkins Frozen Meatloaf
		  with Portobello
		  Mushroom Gravy
		
		Net Carbs: 7g; FV: 4g
			4–6 oz chicken
			1 cup broccoli florets
			1 Tbsp olive oil
			2 cups mixed greens
			2 Tbsp creamy Italian
			  dressing
			
			Net Carbs: 4.5g; FV: 4.3g
				Atkins Frozen Chicken and
				  Broccoli Alfredo
				½ *cup cantaloupe*
				  cubes
				
				Net Carbs: 10.9g; FV: 5g

	Total Net Carbs: 29.3g
	Total Net Carbs from
	  FV: 12.7g
		Total Net Carbs: 30g
		Total Net Carbs from
		  FV: 12.6g
			Total Net Carbs: 29.1g
			Total Net Carbs from
			  FV: 12.1g
				Total Net Carbs: 29.8g
				Total Net Carbs from
				  FV: 15.6g

Enjoy Atkins Endulge Treats for dessert if Net Carb consumption allows!

Friday	Saturday	Sunday
1 cup baby spinach	Atkins Frozen Tex-Mex	2 eggs
1 small tomato	Scramble	2 cups baby spinach
½ avocado	*½ cup raspberries*	1 Tbsp olive oil
1 oz Monterey Jack		½ bell pepper
cheese		1 oz Monterey Jack cheese
25 almonds		*⅓ cup cantaloupe cubes*
Net Carbs: 8.2g; FV: 5.3g	**Net Carbs: 8.4g; FV: 3g**	**Net Carbs: 10.1g; FV: 5.3g**
2 oz Cheddar cheese	Atkins Advantage Caramel	1 stalk celery
1 small tomato	Chocolate Nut Roll Bar	1 oz Cheddar cheese
2 Tbsp vinaigrette	15 walnut halves	
Net Carbs: 3.6g; FV: 2.5g	**Net Carbs: 5.1g; FV: 0g**	**Net Carbs: 1.4g; FV: 1g**
Atkins Frozen Roast	1 6 oz canned tuna or	Atkins Advantage
Turkey Tenders with	fish filet	Chocolate Peanut
Herb Pan Gravy	2 Tbsp mayonnaise or	Butter Bar
	tartar sauce	20 walnut halves
	1 stalk celery	*½ cup raspberries*
	¼ cup chopped bell	
	pepper	
	1 small tomato	
Net Carbs: 6g; FV: 4g	**Net Carbs: 5g; FV: 5g**	**Net Carbs: 8.2g; FV: 0g**
Atkins Advantage	Atkins Advantage Vanilla	½ cup chopped bell
Caramel Chocolate	Shake	pepper
Peanut Nougat Bar	25 almonds	2 Tbsp ranch dressing
5 large strawberries		
Net Carbs: 8.1g; FV: 0g	**Net Carbs: 3.8g; FV: 0g**	**Net Carbs: 2.9g; FV: 2.2g**
4–6 oz ham or pork chop	4 oz steak or hamburger	Atkins Frozen Crustless
1 cup broccoli	1 small tomato	Chicken Pot Pie
1 cup mixed greens	½ avocado	25 almonds
2 Tbsp creamy Italian	½ small onion, sliced	
dressing		
10 walnut halves		
Net Carbs: 4.6g; FV: 2.9g	**Net Carbs: 6.4g; FV: 6.4g**	**Net Carbs: 7.8g; FV: 4g**
Total Net Carbs: 30.5g	**Total Net Carbs: 28.7g**	**Total Net Carbs: 30.4g**
Total Net Carbs from	**Total Net Carbs from**	**Total Net Carbs from**
FV: 14.7g	**FV: 14.4g**	**FV: 12.5g**

WEEK 3 AND BEYOND IN PHASE 2

Assuming that you've already added nuts and seeds and then berries and the like, as discussed previously, your next move would be to introduce foods on the next rung of the Carb Ladder. These additional dairy products include whole-milk yogurt or Greek yogurt (not the flavored or low-fat kind), cottage cheese, and ricotta. You can also have small portions of whole milk. In some cases, you'll be swapping out other foods (replacing Cheddar cheese, for example, with yogurt) to keep carbs in line. After additional dairy products come legumes, and finally tomato and tomato juice cocktail, as well as more lemon and/or lime juice. (See page 113 to review these rungs of the Carb Ladder.)

To modify the earlier meal plans to make them suitable for 35, 40, and 45 grams of Net Carbs, follow these guidelines:

Additional dairy rung: Reintroduce these foods in portions of roughly 5 grams of Net Carbs. For example:

½ cup cottage cheese	4.1 grams Net Carbs
½ cup ricotta cheese	4 grams Net Carbs
¼ cup buttermilk	3.3 grams Net Carbs
¼ cup whole milk	2.9 grams Net Carbs
½ cup whole-milk Greek yogurt (plain, unsweetened)	4.5 grams Net Carbs
½ cup whole-milk yogurt (plain, unsweetened)	5.3 grams Net Carbs

Legumes rung: Reintroduce these foods in portions of roughly 5 grams of Net Carbs. For example:

2 tablespoons cooked chickpeas	5.5 grams Net Carbs
¼ cup cooked lentils	4 grams Net Carbs
2 tablespoons cooked navy beans	5 grams Net Carbs

¼ cup cooked split green peas	6.3 grams Net Carbs
½ cup shelled edamame (green soybeans)	3 grams Net Carbs
3 tablespoons black bean dip	4.5 grams Net Carbs
3 tablespoons hummus	4.5 grams Net Carbs

Tomato and lemon/lime juice rung: Reintroduce these foods in portions of roughly 5 grams of Net Carbs. You can also increase lemon or lime juice from 2 to 4 tablespoons a day.

4 tablespoons lemon juice	4 grams Net Carbs
4 tablespoons lime juice	4.8 grams Net Carbs
½ cup tomato juice	4.0 grams Net Carbs
½ cup tomato-vegetable juice cocktail	4.5 grams Net Carbs

Check the Atkins Carb Counter for other options.

However, as you seek your threshold for carb intake while continuing to shed pounds, known as your carb balance, your daily Net Carb intake may level off well before you transition to Phase 3 (Fine-Tuning). If you have a low carb tolerance, you may choose to experiment with adding some or all of these foods without increasing your daily carb intake or by doing so very slowly.

PHASE 2 SNACKS PDQ

One way to segue into Ongoing Weight Loss is to keep your meals similar to those you ate in Phase 1, but now have snacks that incorporate Phase 2 foods. All Atkins bars and shakes are now acceptable, and you can certainly continue to have your favorites coded for Phase 1. Following are some other snacks you can put together in minutes if you have the fixings in the fridge and pantry. They're also portable. Pop them in an insulated bag with a freezer pack and take them to work or wherever.

- Cottage cheese and berries
- Hummus with radishes or jicama sticks
- Celery sticks stuffed with almond or peanut butter
- Tomato juice with a slice of Cheddar
- Greek yogurt, blueberries, and a packet of sweetener
- Greek yogurt mixed with no-sugar-added salsa, with soy chips
- Sliced avocado on a small low-carb pita bread
- Chopped almonds mixed with half an Atkins bar cut in cubes
- Prosciutto wrapped around cantaloupe slices
- Provolone wrapped around honeydew melon slices
- Small low-carb tortilla with black bean dip and a tomato slice
- Cooked and shelled edamame drizzled with olive oil

MAKE IT EASY

Mascarpone is an ultra-rich and spreadable Italian cheese that makes quick and simple snacks, both savory and sweet. Mix it with mustard or anchovies and serve with raw veggies. It takes on a whole different personality as a snack or dessert when you serve it with berries.

FIND YOUR PERSONAL CARB BALANCE

In Phase 1 (Kick-Start), you, your significant other, your boss, and your great-aunt Hilda can all eat the same amount of carbs and a fixed number of foods and pretty reliably shave off some excess weight. It's the rare individual who doesn't convert to burning primarily fat in the first week of Atkins. Phase 2 (Balancing) is a different story. Whether you're a fast loser or slow loser, in this phase you'll get a grasp on your own metabolism. This understanding will be invaluable as you move toward a permanent way of eating.

There's tremendous variation in how many carbs individuals can consume while continuing to lose weight. (The same applies to maintaining weight, as we'll discuss in Chapter 8.) An active young man might be able to put away 70 grams of Net Carbs a day (or even more) and keep shedding pounds. Meanwhile, a sedentary menopausal woman might hover around 40 grams or even less. Once you understand how sensitive your metabolism is to carbs in general and to certain foods in particular, you'll be armed with the information you need to tailor your progress up the Carb Ladder accordingly. Once more, your personal carb balance is the number of grams of Net Carbs you can consume while continuing to lose weight, feel good, and remain in control of your appetite. This number usually rises as you get closer to your goal.

TROUBLESHOOTING

As you continue to move up the Carb Ladder slowly but deliberately, your weight loss will slow and almost certainly not proceed like clock-work. Both are normal. A loss of 2 or 3 pounds a week might be a rea-sonable expectation for your age, weight, and other factors. However, some weeks you may pare off just a single pound or so, or even a big fat zero. Bottom line: be patient. If your weight loss stalls for several weeks, you may have exceeded your carb tolerance or you may have hit a plateau. How can you tell the difference? And what do you do to reignite fat burning? Let's start with the second question.

STALLED? WHAT'S THE PROBLEM?

Before you panic and jump to the conclusion that you'll never lose an-other pound or that you'll never get above, say, 45 grams of Net Carbs a day, ask yourself these questions.

- Are you counting (not estimating) grams of Net Carbs?
- Are you eating any inappropriate foods?
- Are you supersizing portions?
- Are you overdoing it with berries and/or low-carb products?
- Are you finding certain foods you can't eat in moderation?

- Are you adding additional food, meaning that you're eating more, rather than swapping out other foods (edamame for green beans, for example) to maintain the amount of food?
- Are you eating more than 6 ounces of protein at each meal?
- Have you added all Phase 2 acceptable foods at the same time?
- Have you started drinking wine or beer or using sugar-filled mixers?

Assuming that these queries merit some yes responses, it's time to make one or more modifications to get back on track.

- *Write it down.* Carb creep is all too common as you start to re-introduce certain foods. Enter your food choices, amounts, and Net Carb counts in your journal. You may well be consuming more carbs than you think you are.
- *Play hide and seek.* Look for carbs you may have neglected to count, such as in cream, lemon juice, and even acceptable sweeteners (reminder: count 1 gram of Net Carbs per packet). Also be vigilant about reading labels to ferret out hidden carbs in sauces, condiments, and other processed foods.
- *Abstain for now.* Drinking alcohol could be interfering with fat burning. Eliminate it, as well as any trigger foods.
- *Check your calories.* Although there's no need to count calories on a daily basis, a woman consuming more than 1,800 calories or a man consuming more than 2,200 may simply be eating too much.

If you're not actually on a plateau, you should see weight loss resume once you make the appropriate modifications.

A PLATEAU CALLS FOR PATIENCE

A plateau is defined as an inexplicable pause in weight loss for one month or longer that's not the result of dietary misdemeanors or lifestyle changes. It can happen at any time after you shed the first "easy" pounds, but it is increasingly likely as you approach your goal weight. For inexplicable reasons, your body simply slows down and "refuses" to lose any more weight for a while. Infuriating? Of course. Permanent? Fortunately not. A plateau usually yields to certain strategies, including temporarily reducing your daily carb intake. If you're at, say, 35 grams of Net Carbs a day and hit a plateau, you can cut back by 10 grams and likely some excess pounds will budge. You might even need to go down another 5 grams to 20 grams, which will almost certainly reboot weight loss. Once you're losing again, you can gradually start to increase the carbs.

One possibility is that you've stumbled upon your carb tolerance level without realizing it. If cutting back on carbs doesn't do the trick, pretty much the only thing to do is wait out the plateau, although adding regular physical activity if you haven't already done so may also bust it. It will certainly help you maintain your weight and handle the stress the plateau occasions. (See "Nowhere to Go," below, if you plateau while following the Fast Track.)

Although it sounds counterintuitive, some people have found that slightly increasing their carb intake or adding a new acceptable food kick-starts weight loss again. Patience is definitely a virtue when it comes to a plateau. As you'll remember from Charity W.'s story (page 48), she waited out an eight-week period of no weight loss!

NOWHERE TO GO

If you're following the Fast Track by remaining in Phase 1, busting a plateau is challenging. When you're consuming just 20 daily grams of Net Carbs for an extended period of time, it may be tempting to drop below 20 grams a day, but it's not healthful to sacrifice foundation vegetables to do so. You simply have to hang in there. Moreover, overly restricting choices in Phase 1 can make the program too difficult for the long haul.

IDENTIFY AND AVOID TRIGGER FOODS

If you can't seem to eat just a few nuts, you already know what a trigger food is: it's any food, whether an acceptable one such as nuts or an unacceptable one such as chocolate chip cookies, that you can't eat in moderate portions and which may make you hungry for other foods as well. Once you have one (or a handful), you can't stop eating until the box or bag or jar is empty. The best way to deal with unacceptable trigger foods is to banish them from the house if possible. With Atkins-friendly foods such as peanuts, measure out portions ahead of time to avoid overeating.

The urge to binge is a clear indicator that you may have exceeded your carb threshold. If you're eating too many carbs, fat burning ceases and with it the empowerment of appetite suppression. Bingeing isn't just a matter of eating more carbs than you should; it's being totally out of control, often as a result of eating a trigger food. Eating a second 1-ounce bag of almonds is an indiscretion; snarfing down a pint of rocky road ice cream is a binge. The only solution to such overindulgence is to stop it before it occurs.

In addition to not going too long between meals, always having acceptable foods in the house, and not shopping while you're hungry, these tips should help head off the urge to binge:

- Call your buddy (or a sympathetic family member or friend) for help *before* you succumb.
- Don't eat in front of the television or computer, at the movies, or in any other place where it's easy for hand-to-mouth movements to go on automatic pilot. (The exception to this rule is if you're having a single portion-controlled Atkins meal or bar.)
- Have substitute foods on hand. If a chocolate chip cookie can send you off the deep end, an Atkins Advantage bar should tame your chocolate lust.

FREQUENTLY ASKED QUESTIONS

Q. How do I get back on track after an "indiscretion"?
A. First of all, don't beat yourself up. We all have moments of weakness, and maybe that plate of french fries your friend was eating was more than you could resist. Second, don't play the game of "Well, since I've already messed up, I might as well go whole hog." For the rest of the day eat appropriately. Don't wait until tomorrow to get back on the wagon.

Q. What's carb creep?
A. Without realizing it, as you gradually add back foods, you may be consuming far more carbs than you think you are. This can make you complacent about your intake until your weight loss stalls. Once again, tracking your carbs and portion sizes should help you avoid carb creep.

Q. Why have my cravings returned?
A. Usually cravings vanish by the end of the first week on Induction when you convert to burning primarily fat for energy. There are several reasons they may return. Women sometimes experience cravings a few days before their menstrual period. Going too long between meals or adding foods such as dairy products or peanuts may stimulate cravings. Stress can also destabilize blood sugar, triggering cravings for comfort foods. Adding a bit more fat, in the form of olives, half an avocado, or some cream cheese in a celery stick, can help you feel more satisfied, minimizing cravings.

Q. Do I have to reintroduce all Phase 2 acceptable foods?
A. Of course not. If you don't like yogurt or chickpeas or tomato juice, so be it. Or if a whole rung on the Carb Ladder holds no appeal for you, just skip it. There's still plenty of variety inherent in the whole foods you can eat on Atkins.

Q. Why is my weight loss erratic?

A. As I've discussed with regard to plateaus, your body has its own schedule and won't share it with anyone. The important thing is to follow the program faithfully and the pounds will come off. Again, adding exercise helps some people lose weight, but not everyone. Be *sure* to take your measurements weekly. If you've lost inches, the scale is bound to catch up.

Q. Why have I regained some of the weight I lost?

A. The reason I recommend that you *not* weigh yourself daily is that your weight can vary by as much as 5 pounds even within a day. As long as you're following the program, you should see some weight loss every week or so, unless you're on a plateau. If you stayed on track but gained a pound or two since the previous week, you're probably retaining water or are constipated.

WHEN TO SAY GOODBYE TO PHASE 2

There are two big questions you'll face in the Balancing phase. The first we've alluded to throughout this chapter: "How do I find my personal carb balance, my threshold for consuming carbs while losing weight?" The answer? By trial and error! You'll gradually increase your daily Net Carb count. If weight loss levels off, you'll cut back by 5 grams of Net Carbs to see if it gets going again. When it does, you'll add another 5 grams, and so forth. You'll want to go as high as you can as long as weight loss continues, albeit more slowly than before, and you continue to feel good and in control of cravings. There is no right number, only the one that feels right to you and which you can maintain without too much effort.

The second, and related, question is, "When should I transition to Phase 3?" If you've lost weight steadily and are now only about 10 pounds from your goal weight, the answer is simple: now! Why? Because your long-term goal is to find a sustainable way of eating. And with 10 pounds to go, you have enough time to try to reintroduce the remaining carb foods. If you aren't yet 10 pounds from your goal, the answer is that it depends, just like when you were deciding when to transition to Phase 2.

In that case, ask yourself which of these three scenarios describes you:

1. You've reached a daily intake of about 50 grams of Net Carbs, have introduced Phase 2 foods, and continue to slim down without experiencing cravings and unreasonable hunger. If so, feel free to transition to Phase 3 now if you're eager for more variety in your meals. If you stall out there, you can always return to Phase 2 to reboot weight loss.

2. You still have more than 10 pounds to shed and are stalled in your weight-loss progress and/or experiencing cravings and extreme hunger before meals. By all means, stay in this phase until the cravings and hunger have vanished.

3. Although you lost weight in Phase 1, your progress in this phase has been frustrating, and some Phase 2 foods are creating cravings and undue hunger. You may have even gained a few pounds. You may be extraordinarily sensitive to carbs and may have reached your carb tolerance at 30 or 35 grams of Net Carbs. Follow the advice above, be patient, and ramp up your activity level if possible.

Now turn the page to meet Troy G., whose life seemed to be falling apart eleven years ago as he faced his excess weight, a serious gastrointestinal problem, and bankruptcy. Today, he's a lean ultra-marathon runner who knows that carb loading is not the only way to run a race. Read his story to get inspired to add fitness to your weight-loss program. In the next chapter, we'll move on to Phase 3, Pre-Maintenance, where you'll achieve your goal weight and begin the dress rehearsal for a lifetime of slimness.

ON THE RIGHT TRACK FOR GOOD

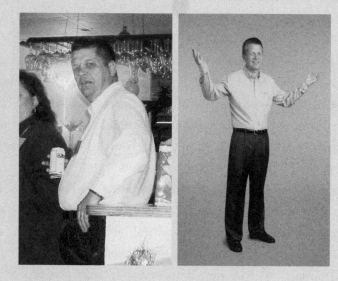

VITAL STATS

Daily Net Carb intake: 60–70
  grams

Age: 50

Height: 5'11"

Before weight: 233 pounds

After weight: 163 pounds

Weight lost: 70 pounds

Troy G.'s life was in free fall. At age thirty-nine, he was an overweight couch potato confronting his own health issues, and concerned about his wife, who had become partially disabled. Troy had lost his job and some business deals had gone wrong. The couple declared bankruptcy and their home was in foreclosure. In the midst of these troubles, Troy started Atkins, shed his excess weight within six months, and started running. Before long, his health was restored and he could boast a BMI of about 21. A new job took the family to College Station, Texas. Eleven years later, Troy remains committed to the Atkins lifestyle. Let's hear how he turned his life around.

I was always a skinny kid. When I played baseball in high school, I worked out and took supplements to bulk up. But in college I started living on pizza and beer, and after graduation I continued to live on junk food and my job as a software developer and programmer was a sedentary one. That skinny kid had become a heavy man. With everything out of control, I decided that the only things that I *could* control were my weight and my health.

I had lost weight before. After surgery to deal with diverticulitis, I was put on a liquid diet. I lost weight, but of course I regained it when I went back to eating solid food. One day when I was at my heaviest, I was playing peewee tackle football with my younger son, who was about six at the time. I caught a pass and all I had to do was run a few yards to make the touchdown. Instead, I fell down. My son said, "Dad, would you play on the other team now?" That was my inspiration to be a role model for him by showing that you shouldn't give up on your goals.

I'd done what I thought was Atkins a couple of times before, but I was just cutting carbs without knowing what I was doing. This time I read *The New Atkins for a New You*, and my wife and I did Atkins together. We started with Induction and followed it to the letter. Although I've never been much for vegetables, I ate as much as I could, but can't say that I ever developed a taste for broccoli! I lost a pound and sometimes even two each day and never hit a plateau.

After three or four months I'd found how many carbs I could consume and keep losing weight, and within six months I was down 70 pounds. I was feeling so much better and more energetic that I decided to take up running. After a few months I began to enter 5-kilometer races and then worked up to half marathons and finally marathons. This was all within a year of starting Atkins. Now I'm proud to call myself an ultra-marathon runner, having completed twenty-one marathons, as well as a dozen ultra-marathons (thirty-one miles or greater). I've even run seventy miles in a twenty-four-hour period to match my weight loss of 70 pounds.

For many years I followed my low-carb lifestyle, but I was taking the conventional path of carb loading before a race. I did okay, but I was always hitting the wall. After a marathon, I would feel like I had the ultimate hangover, but I continued to train that way. Then I did some research on how dietary fat provides more sustained energy than carbs and found that I could run on a low-carb regimen. I'd been training that way for a couple of months and decided to try it on a seventy-mile celebratory run. I was able to do it by drinking Atkins shakes and taking breaks to rest or walk.

I was still not totally convinced that fat loading was the way to go, but in the next marathon I tried it, and it was the easiest one I'd ever run. I usually hit the wall at the twenty-mile point, but this time I was able to actually run faster after that point than during the earlier part of the race.

My lucky number is now 70. It's my proof that you can take control of your life, that you can feel good about yourself and endure anything that is thrown at you. And 70 is also my personal proof that the Atkins lifestyle does work, not only for losing weight, but also for successfully preparing for endurance events.

I have to say that I've developed a totally different outlook on life. At forty years old, I finally learned to distinguish between what I could control and focus on that, and to let go of what I couldn't control. The Atkins lifestyle helped me gain control of my life. And as far as football goes, when my kids began their next peewee tackle season after I'd lost the 70 pounds, the coach didn't recognize me. And no one was suggesting I play for the other team!

Note: Troy has written a Nook ebook, *Endurance 70*, dedicated to the late Dr. Atkins, about his experience as an endurance athlete. It is available at bn.com.

CHAPTER 7

THE FINISH LINE IS IN SIGHT

You're probably now just 10 pounds from your goal weight, which you'll achieve in Phase 3, Pre-Maintenance (Fine-Tuning). Bravo! You've worked hard, been patient, and deserve the reward you're closing in on: a slim, healthy new you. I won't say the end is near, because reaching your goal weight is actually just the beginning of your new lifestyle. And if you've opted to begin this phase with more than 10 pounds to go, you can still begin to broaden your food choices, although it may take you a bit longer to reach your goal weight.

TIME TO FINE-TUNE

When you transitioned to Phase 2 (Balancing), the trick was to go as slow as molasses (yes, I know it's an added sugar)—that is, gradually and deliberately. You'll do the same again as you see how much you can raise your daily Net Carb intake while exploring the final three rungs of the Carb Ladder (see page 151) in Phase 3 (Fine-Tuning). They include foods with the highest carb counts: fruits other than berries, cherries, and melon; starchy vegetables; and whole grains, building on the foods lower on the Carb Ladder that you've already been eating. You might be able to eat all these "new" foods; another possibility, however, is that your metabolism may be able to handle only some of them—or small amounts. Or you may find that you can eat them rarely or not at all.

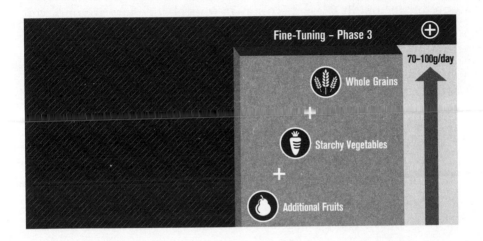

In this phase you'll come to understand how your body reacts to these foods in terms of slowing weight loss, halting it altogether, or prompting cravings or unreasonable hunger. All this is part of continuing to explore your tolerance for carbs while continuing to *lose* weight (what we call your personal carb balance) and then ultimately finding your slightly higher tolerance for carbs as you *maintain* weight loss.

PHASE 3 GUIDELINES

As you've already learned, the last thing you want to do is rush to add back all the Phase 3 foods that you've been missing. After all, fruit, bread, potatoes, cereals, and grains are probably among the culprits that got you in trouble to begin with. Add them back all at once and you'll almost certainly stall your fat-burning engine. But that's no reason to hang out in Phase 2. To stay in control, inch forward until you discover how far you can go, and you'll know exactly what you can and cannot eat. Then make it your permanent way of eating to eliminate the struggles with weight you've experienced in the past. Much of the advice on how to succeed in Phase 3 will sound familiar, because it's the natural extension of Phase 2.

- Continue to consume a minimum of 12–15 grams of Net Carbs in the form of foundation vegetables, avoid foods with added sugar, have eight glasses of water or other acceptable fluids each day, and go no longer than three or four waking hours without eating, spreading out your carb intake across meals and snacks.

- Reintroduce new food groups one by one, following the Carb Ladder. Depending on your metabolism and weight-loss goal, this may be at weekly, biweekly, or even longer intervals.

- Add back carbohydrate foods within each rung of the Carb Ladder one by one. For example, reintroduce apples but gauge their impact, if any, for a couple of days before adding oranges.

- Increase your overall Net Carb intake in 10-gram increments (if you've been losing weight relatively easily) or 5-gram increments (if weight loss has slowed). Make these increases no more frequently than once a week; you can also do so every two weeks, or even less frequently.

- Continue to log your daily Net Carb intake in your journal, also noting any "new" foods so that you can ascertain if any of them are stalling your progress.
- Once you reach your goal weight, remain at that level of Net Carb intake for one month to ensure you can maintain it.
- Continue to weigh and measure yourself weekly.

Now let's review the acceptable Phase 3 foods, understanding that you may not be able to reintroduce all of them.

ACCEPTABLE PHASE 3 FOODS

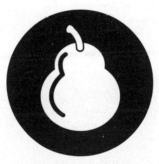

OTHER FRUITS

Although legumes are acceptable in OWL, you may not have added them back yet. If so, do that before moving to fruit. (See page 113 for suggestions.) On the other hand, if you're not big on lentils and other beans, simply skip them. As with the earlier lists of acceptable foods, the following include just a few representative foods on each rung of the Carb Ladder. Refer to the Atkins Carb Counter for more complete lists with serving sizes and Net Carb counts. Use the printed version available from Atkins, download it from atkins.com, or use the Atkins mobile app.

As with the berries, cherries, and melon that you reintroduced in OWL, have these higher-carb fruits in small quantities, starting with one at a time and only once a day. Have fresh or frozen (unsweetened) fruit or fruit canned in water or juice rather than syrup. Avoid fruit juice and sweetened applesauce. Tropical fruits such as banana, mango, and plantain are considerably higher in carbs than other fruits, so wait on them until you see how you tolerate other fruits. As long as they're made without added sugar, small portions of jelly, jam, preserves, and fruit preserves made from Phase 3 fruits are also acceptable. (See "Low-Carb Resources" on page 212 for sources.)

- Apples
- Apricots
- Grapes
- Grapefruit
- Kiwis
- Oranges
- Papayas
- Peaches or nectarines
- Pears
- Plums
- Pomegranates
- Watermelon

MAKE IT EASY

Save time by picking up packaged cut-up fresh fruit in the produce section. Divide the contents into appropriate portions to eat at home or take to work.

THE SCOOP ON SUGAR: FRESH VERSUS DRIED FRUIT

The process of drying fruit evaporates the water and concentrates the sugar content. Therefore, the amount of fresh fruit considered a single serving is not the same as for a single serving of dried fruit. Compare the carb counts in the table below—dried fruits are shown in italics—and you'll see why they should be consumed in moderation.

FRUIT	AMOUNT AND TYPE	GRAMS OF NET CARBS
Apple	½ fresh	7.9
Apple	*1 ounce freeze-dried*	*23*
Banana	1 small fresh	20.4
Banana	*1 ounce freeze-dried*	*23*
Currants	¼ cup fresh	6.0
Currants	*2 tablespoons dried*	*12.1*
Grapes, Concord	½ cup	7.5
Raisins	*1 tablespoon*	*6.8*
Mango	½ cup fresh	11.1
Mango	*1 piece, freeze-dried*	*21*
Papaya	½ cup fresh	6.6
Papaya	*1 strip, dried*	*12.2*

GO EASY ON FRUIT

Reintroduce fruit slowly and in small amounts, particularly if you've been craving it until now. To stay in control:

- Swap one serving of berries or melon for a serving of higher-carb fruits.
- Have no more than two fruit servings (including berries) a day.
- Always accompany fruit with some fat or protein.
- Start with the lower-carb fruits in this category, such as papayas, peaches, plums, or tangerines.

- Go "halfsies" by sharing an apple, pear, grapefruit, or papaya with a family member, or save the other half for tomorrow.
- Garnish your breakfast eggs with ½ cup grapes or orange sections, or add them to a salad.
- Eat fruits such as bananas, pears, papayas, and mangos *before* they're very ripe, to minimize the impact on blood sugar.
- Combine higher-carb fruits in a fruit salad with lower-carb berries and/or melon.

STARCHY VEGETABLES

You've been eating plenty of foundation vegetables in the first two phases of the New Atkins Diet. After reintroducing other fruits, it's time to try to reintroduce the rest of the vegetable family. Like foundation veggies, these roots, tubers, and other veggies are high in fiber and antioxidants; however, they're higher in carbs. A half cup of baked acorn squash, for example, tallies 7.8 grams of Net Carbs; half a sweet potato and half a baked white potato contain 12.1 and 10.5 grams, respectively. Comparable servings of some tropical vegetables such as cassava (yuca), taro, and yautia are significantly higher in carbs. Among the choices are:

- Beets
- Carrots

- Corn on (or off) the cob
- Jerusalem artichokes
- Peas
- Parsnips
- Potatoes, sweet and white
- Rutabagas
- Winter squash
- Yams

CURB THOSE CARBS

To enjoy some new veggies without going overboard, try these ideas on for size:

- Have carrots raw instead of cooked, as cooking raises the carb count.
- Add ¼ cup grated carrot to tuna or chicken salad.
- Add grated carrots to cabbage slaw.
- Steam potatoes and cauliflower and mash together to mute the carb impact of potatoes.
- Make succotash with equal portions of frozen corn and edamame (instead of higher-carb lima beans).
- Roast a single cut-up potato or sweet potato with several foundation vegetables.
- Instead of squash soup, combine one part squash with twice as much pumpkin, which is actually a foundation veggie.
- Sauté ¼ cup peas with sliced scallions and thinly sliced lettuce.

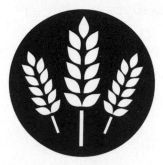

WHOLE GRAINS

Occupying the top rung of the Carb Ladder, grains are the last whole-food group to reintroduce. Not everyone can tolerate grains and products made with them, so proceed with caution. And don't confuse refined grains such as white flour and white rice with whole grains. Baked goods, including bread, pita, tortillas, crackers, and cereals, made with refined grains remain on the "avoid" list indefinitely (with the exception of low-carb products). Such products made with whole grains are acceptable, but the Net Carb counts may vary greatly from one product to another. Here are some of the more common whole grains:

- Barley
- Cornmeal and hominy
- Couscous, whole-wheat
- Kasha (buckwheat groats)
- Whole-wheat flour, wheat berries, bulgur, and cracked wheat
- Millet
- Oat bran and old-fashioned or steel-cut oatmeal (not instant)
- Quinoa
- Rice, brown, red, or wild

In Phase 3 you can also increase your daily intake of whole milk to ½ cup, but continue to steer clear of low-fat milk and other low-fat dairy products. You also can experiment with low-carb products that have up to 9 grams of Net Carbs per serving. For an extended list of foods in these three rungs of the Carb Ladder, along with serving sizes and Net Carb gram counts, see the Atkins Carb Counter.

A LITTLE GOES A LONG WAY

When adding grains back into your diet, the best approach is to use very small portions, treating them as a garnish or a small component of a dish, rather than the star attraction. Instead of a conventional serving of a grain:

- Top a tossed salad with a little cooked wild rice, wheat berries, or other whole grain.
- Combine equal proportions of cooked oatmeal, oat bran, and chopped nuts for a relatively low-carb hot breakfast.
- Swap the proportions of a grain salad by using a small amount of cracked wheat, quinoa, or kasha and plenty of chopped parsley, mint, scallions, cucumber, and tomatoes.
- Mix a little cooked brown or wild rice into a stir-fry with zucchini, red bell peppers, and leftover chicken or beef.

FIND YOUR OWN PACE IN PHASE 3

As in the second phase, how individuals navigate the increase in food choices and grams of Net Carbs varies greatly. If you're still losing reliably each week, you may be able to move up in 10-gram increments and reintroduce all the food groups, one after another. Or you may need to use 5-gram increments some weeks and hang back at other times. If your tolerance for carbs is low and your weight loss has proceeded slowly or in fits and starts, it may take you considerably longer to introduce new foods. Someone with a high metabolism might have reached his or her goal weight and been able to reintroduce all rungs of the Carb Ladder after a month in Phase 3. Someone with a slow metabolism, in contrast, might take three months or more to get there and never reach the top of the Carb Ladder. Don't move to a higher carb count or add a new food group if you stop losing. Again, not everyone will be able to reintroduce all Phase 3 foods, or it could take several months to do so without stalling weight loss or provoking cravings and undue hunger.

WEEK-AT-A-GLANCE MEAL PLANS FOR PHASE 3

The following three plans continue to progressively build upon one of the original meal plans, making it easy to reintroduce foods from the final three rungs of the Carb Ladder (see page 151). If you have reached these Net Carb daily levels but not reintroduced all the rungs of the Carb Ladder, your carb intake may differ from these sample meal plans. However, the three plans do illustrate how to gradually and progressively modify your intake as you climb the Carb Ladder and approach your goal weight.

WEEK-AT-A-GLANCE MEAL PLAN AT 50 GRAMS OF NET CARBS A DAY

Continuing to evolve from the original Phase 1 meal plan, this plan assumes you've already reintroduced nuts and seeds, berries and other low-carb fruits, more dairy products, legumes, and tomato juice. It adds back other fruits, swapping one serving of berries for higher-carb fruit, one at a time. As before, substitutions and additions are small and incremental, to make the transition as simple as possible. Easy suggestions for how to add back these foods are indicated in boldface italic type in the meal plan on page 162. Substitute other fruits for the items listed, if you prefer, using the Atkins Carb Counter to stay within the Net Carb guidelines.

WEEK AT-A-GLANCE MEAL PLAN AT 60 GRAMS OF NET CARBS A DAY

The next rung on the Carb Ladder is reflected in the next evolution of the meal plan shown on page 164, with a starchy vegetable sometimes taking the place of a foundation vegetable. Simple suggestions for how to add them back appear in boldface italic type on the plan. Substitute other starchy vegetables with a comparable Net Carb count for those listed if you prefer, referring to the Atkins Carb Counter. However, remember that not everyone will be able to include starchy vegetables or this level of carb intake.

WEEK-AT-A-GLANCE MEAL PLAN AT 70 GRAMS OF NET CARBS A DAY

The last meal plan (on page 166) reintroduces whole grains, the final rung of the Carb Ladder, building upon the earlier plans. Simple suggestions for how to add these foods back are indicated in boldface italic type in the meal plan on page 166. Not all people will be able to include whole grains or this level of carb intake. If you find that you can go higher than 70 daily grams of Net Carbs, adjust the meal plan accordingly.

Atkins Phase 3 (Fine-Tuning) Meal Plan at 50g NC/day

	Monday	Tuesday	Wednesday	Thursday
BREAKFAST	2 eggs ¼ cup chopped onion 1 tsp olive oil 1 oz Cheddar cheese ½ cup tomato juice **Net Carbs: 8.5g; FV: 7.5g**	Atkins Advantage Peanut Butter Granola Bar 5 large strawberries **Net Carbs: 8.1g; FV: 0g**	Atkins Frozen Farmhouse-Style Sausage Scramble ⅓ cup cantaloupe cubes ½ cup Greek yogurt **Net Carbs: 13.6g; FV: 1g**	4 oz steak or hamburger 1 tsp olive oil ½ cup chopped bell pepper ¼ cup chopped onion 1 oz Cheddar cheese **Net Carbs: 5.6g; FV: 5.3g**
SNACK	Atkins Advantage Vanilla Shake 10 almonds 5 large strawberries **Net Carbs: 7.2g; FV: 0g**	1 small tomato 1 oz Monterey Jack cheese **Net Carbs: 2.7g; FV: 2.5g**	¾ cup sliced bell pepper ¼ cup hummus 10 walnut halves **Net Carbs: 9.1g; FV: 2.8g**	Atkins Advantage Milk Chocolate Delight Shake ½ *medium apple* **Net Carbs: 10.5g; FV: 0g**
LUNCH	Atkins Frozen Crustless Chicken Pot Pie ½ *medium pear* **Net Carbs: 16g; FV: 4g**	4–6 oz chicken 1 small tomato 1 cup mixed greens ½ avocado 2 Tbsp ranch dressing ⅓ cup cooked lentils **Net Carbs: 13.9g; FV: 5.1g**	Atkins Frozen Beef Merlot ½ *medium pear* **Net Carbs: 17g; FV: 4g**	4–6 oz ham or pork chop ⅓ cup cooked lentils 1 cup baby spinach ½ avocado 1 Tbsp ranch dressing **Net Carbs: 11.6g; FV: 2.8g**
SNACK	Atkins Advantage Coconut Almond Delight Bar 10 almonds **Net Carbs: 4.1g; FV: 0g**	1 stalk celery 1 oz Cheddar cheese 20 almonds **Net Carbs: 3.6g; FV: 1g**	Atkins Advantage Café Caramel Shake 25 almonds **Net Carbs: 4.8g; FV: 0g**	1 small tomato 2 Tbsp vinaigrette 25 almonds **Net Carbs: 5.7g; FV: 2.5g**
DINNER	4–6 oz canned tuna or fish filet 2 cups mixed greens ½ avocado ¼ cup garbanzo beans 2 Tbsp vinaigrette 1 cup broccoli florets **Net Carbs: 14.1g; FV: 5.6g**	Atkins Frozen Meatloaf with Portobello Mushroom Gravy ½ *medium pear* ½ cup cottage cheese **Net Carbs: 22.1g; FV: 4g**	4–6 oz chicken 1 cup broccoli florets 2 cups mixed greens 2 Tbsp creamy Italian dressing **Net Carbs: 4.5g; FV: 4.3g**	Atkins Frozen Chicken and Broccoli Alfredo ½ cup cantaloupe cubes ½ cup Greek yogurt **Net Carbs: 15.6g; FV: 5g**
	Total Net Carbs: 49.9g **Total Net Carbs from FV: 17.1g**	**Total Net Carbs: 50.4g** **Total Net Carbs from FV: 17g**	**Total Net Carbs: 49.1g** **Total Net Carbs from FV: 12.1g**	**Total Net Carbs: 49g** **Total Net Carbs from FV: 15.6g**

Enjoy Atkins Endulge Treats for dessert if Net Carb consumption allows!

Friday	Saturday	Sunday
1 cup baby spinach 1 small tomato ½ avocado 1 oz Monterey Jack cheese 10 almonds **Net Carbs: 6.5g; FV: 5.3g**	Atkins Frozen Tex-Mex Scramble ½ cup raspberries ½ cup Greek yogurt **Net Carbs: 13.1g; FV: 3g**	2 eggs 2 cups baby spinach 1 tsp olive oil ½ bell pepper 1 oz Monterey Jack cheese ½ cup cantaloupe cubes **Net Carbs: 12g; FV: 5.3g**
1 small tomato ½ cup cottage cheese **Net Carbs: 6.6g; FV: 2.5g**	Atkins Advantage Caramel Chocolate Nut Roll Bar 15 walnut halves **Net Carbs: 5.1g; FV: 0g**	2 stalks celery 1 oz Cheddar cheese ½ cup tomato juice **Net Carbs: 6.7g; FV: 6.4g**
Atkins Frozen Roast Turkey Tenders with Herb Pan Gravy ½ *medium pear* **Net Carbs: 17g; FV: 4g**	4–6 oz canned tuna or fish filet 2 Tbsp mayonnaise or tartar sauce 1 stalk celery ¼ cup chopped bell pepper 1 small tomato **Net Carbs: 5g; FV: 5g**	Atkins Advantage Chocolate Peanut Butter Bar 20 walnut halves **Net Carbs: 4.8g; FV: 0g**
Atkins Advantage Caramel Chocolate Peanut Nougat Bar 5 large strawberries **Net Carbs: 8.1g; FV: 0g**	Atkins Advantage Vanilla Shake 25 almonds ½ *medium pear* **Net Carbs: 14.8g; FV: 0g**	1 cup sliced bell pepper ¼ cup hummus **Net Carbs: 8.7g; FV: 3.7g**
4–6 oz ham or pork chop 1 cup broccoli 1 cup mixed greens ¼ cup garbanzo beans 2 Tbsp creamy Italian dressing 10 walnut halves **Net Carbs: 12.7g; FV: 2.9g**	4 oz steak or hamburger 1 small tomato ½ avocado ½ small onion, sliced ¼ cup cooked lentils **Net Carbs: 12.4g; FV: 6.4g**	Atkins Frozen Crustless Chicken Pot Pie ½ *medium apple* 25 almonds **Net Carbs: 16.3g; FV: 4g**
Total Net Carbs: 50.9g **Total Net Carbs from FV: 14.7g**	**Total Net Carbs: 50.4g** **Total Net Carbs from FV: 14.4g**	**Total Net Carbs: 48.5g** **Total Net Carbs from FV: 19.4g**

Atkins Phase 3 (Fine-Tuning) Meal Plan at 60g NC/day

	Monday	Tuesday	Wednesday	Thursday
BREAKFAST	2 eggs ¼ cup chopped onion 1 tsp olive oil 1 oz Cheddar cheese ½ cup tomato juice Net Carbs: 8.5g; FV: 7.5g	Atkins Advantage Peanut Butter Granola Bar 25 almonds 7 large strawberries Net Carbs: 13g; FV: 0g	Atkins Frozen Farmhouse- Style Sausage Scramble ½ cup cantaloupe cubes ½ cup Greek yogurt Net Carbs: 15.5g; FV: 1g	4 oz steak or hamburger 1 tsp olive oil ½ cup chopped bell pepper ¼ cup chopped onion 1 oz Cheddar cheese Net Carbs: 5.6g; FV: 5.3g
SNACK	Atkins Advantage Vanilla Shake 10 almonds 5 large strawberries Net Carbs: 7.2g; FV: 0g	1 stalk celery 1 oz Monterey Jack cheese ½ cup tomato juice Net Carbs: 5.6g; FV: 5.4g	¾ cup sliced bell pepper ¼ cup hummus 10 walnut halves Net Carbs: 9.1g; FV: 2.8g	Atkins Advantage Milk Chocolate Delight Shake ½ medium apple Net Carbs: 10.5g; FV: 0g
LUNCH	Atkins Frozen Crustless Chicken Pot Pie *½ cup peas* Net Carbs: 12g; FV: 4g	4–6 oz chicken 1 small tomato 2 cups mixed greens ½ avocado 2 Tbsp ranch dressing ⅓ cup cooked lentils 25 almonds Net Carbs: 18g; FV: 6.4g	Atkins Frozen Beef Merlot *½ cup peas* *⅓ cup cooked sliced carrots* Net Carbs: 17.1g; FV: 4g	4–6 oz ham or pork chop ⅓ cup cooked lentils *½ cup peas* *⅓ cup cooked sliced carrots* 1 cup baby spinach ½ avocado 1 Tbsp ranch dressing Net Carbs: 21.3g; FV: 2.8g
SNACK	Atkins Advantage Coconut Almond Delight Bar 10 almonds ½ medium pear Net Carbs: 15.1g; FV: 0g	½ medium apple 1 oz Cheddar cheese Net Carbs: 8.9g; FV: 0g	Atkins Advantage Café Caramel Shake 25 almonds Net Carbs: 4.8g; FV: 0g	1 small tomato 2 Tbsp vinaigrette 25 almonds Net Carbs: 5.7g; FV: 2.5g
DINNER	4–6 oz canned tuna or fish filet 2 cups mixed greens ½ avocado ⅓ cup garbanzo beans 2 Tbsp vinaigrette 1 cup broccoli florets Net Carbs: 16.8g; FV: 5.6g	Atkins Frozen Meatloaf with Portobello Mushroom Gravy *½ cup peas* Net Carbs: 14g; FV: 4g	4–6 oz chicken 1 cup broccoli florets 2 cups mixed greens 2 Tbsp creamy Italian dressing ½ medium pear Net Carbs: 15.5g; FV: 4.3g	Atkins Frozen Chicken and Broccoli Alfredo ½ cup cantaloupe cubes ½ cup Greek yogurt Net Carbs: 15.6g; FV: 5g
	Total Net Carbs: 59.6g Total Net Carbs from FV: 17.1g	Total Net Carbs: 59.5g Total Net Carbs from FV: 15.8g	Total Net Carbs: 62g Total Net Carbs from FV: 12.1g	Total Net Carbs: 58.7g Total Net Carbs from FV: 15.6g

Enjoy Atkins Endulge Treats for dessert if Net Carb consumption allows!

Friday	Saturday	Sunday
1 cup baby spinach	Atkins Frozen Tex-Mex	2 eggs
1 small tomato	Scramble	2 cups baby spinach
½ avocado	½ medium apple	1 tsp olive oil
1 oz Monterey Jack	½ cup Greek yogurt	½ bell pepper
cheese		1 oz Monterey Jack cheese
10 almonds		½ cup cantaloupe cubes
Net Carbs: 6.5g; FV: 5.3g	**Net Carbs: 18.2g; FV: 3g**	**Net Carbs: 12g; FV: 5.3g**
½ medium apple	Atkins Advantage	2 stalks celery
20 almonds	Caramel Chocolate Nut	2 oz Cheddar cheese
	Roll Bar	½ cup tomato juice
Net Carbs: 10.8g; FV: 0g	**Net Carbs: 3g; FV: 0g**	**Net Carbs: 7.1g; FV: 6.4g**
Atkins Frozen Roast	4–6 oz canned tuna or	Atkins Advantage
Turkey Tenders with	fish filet	Chocolate Peanut
Herb Pan Gravy	2 Tbsp mayonnaise or	Butter Bar
⅓ **cup small baked**	tartar sauce	20 walnut halves
potato	2 stalks celery	½ medium pear
	¼ cup chopped bell	
	pepper	
	1 small tomato	
Net Carbs: 14.7g; FV: 4g	**Net Carbs: 6g; FV: 6g**	**Net Carbs: 15.8g; FV: 0g**
Atkins Advantage Caramel	Atkins Advantage Vanilla	1 cup sliced bell pepper
Chocolate Peanut	Shake	¼ cup hummus
Nougat Bar	25 almonds	
10 large strawberries	½ medium pear	
Net Carbs: 13.2g; FV: 0g	**Net Carbs: 14.8g; FV: 0g**	**Net Carbs: 8.7g; FV: 3.7g**
4–6 oz ham or pork chop	4 oz steak or hamburger	Atkins Frozen Crustless
1 cup broccoli	1 medium tomato	Chicken Pot Pie
1 cup mixed greens	½ avocado	½ **cup peas**
⅓ cup garbanzo beans	½ small onion, sliced	½ **cup cooked sliced**
2 Tbsp creamy Italian	⅓ **cup small baked**	**carrots**
dressing	**potato**	
10 walnut halves		
Net Carbs: 15.4g; FV: 2.9g	**Net Carbs: 16g; FV: 7.2g**	**Net Carbs: 16.1g; FV: 4g**
Total Net Carbs: 60.6g	**Total Net Carbs: 58g**	**Total Net Carbs: 59.7g**
Total Net Carbs from	**Total Net Carbs from**	**Total Net Carbs from**
FV: 12.2g	**FV: 16.2g**	**FV: 19.4g**

Atkins Phase 3 (Fine-Tuning) Meal Plan at 70g NC/day

	Monday	Tuesday	Wednesday	Thursday

BREAKFAST	2 eggs
	¼ cup chopped onion
	1 tsp olive oil
	1 oz Cheddar cheese
	½ cup tomato juice
	
	Net Carbs: 8.5g; FV: 7.5g
		Atkins Advantage Peanut
		  Butter Granola Bar
		15 almonds
		½ medium pear
		
		Net Carbs: 15.7g; FV: 0g
			Atkins Frozen Farmhouse-
			  Style Sausage
			  Scramble
			½ cup cantaloupe cubes
			½ cup Greek yogurt
			
			Net Carbs: 15.5g; FV: 1g
				4 oz steak or hamburger
				1 tsp olive oil
				½ cup chopped bell
				  pepper
				¼ cup chopped onion
				1 oz Cheddar cheese
				Net Carbs: 5.6g; FV: 5.3g

SNACK	Atkins Advantage
	  Vanilla Shake
	8 large strawberries
	Net Carbs: 9.2g; FV: 0g
		1 stalk celery
		1 oz Monterey Jack cheese
		½ cup tomato juice
		Net Carbs: 5.6g; FV: 5.4g
			¾ cup sliced bell pepper
			¼ cup hummus
			4 whole wheat crackers
			Net Carbs: 18.6g; FV: 2.8g
				Atkins Advantage Milk
				  Chocolate Delight Shake
				½ medium apple
				Net Carbs: 10.5g; FV: 0g

LUNCH	Atkins Frozen Crustless
	  Chicken Pot Pie
	½ cup peas
	¼ cup brown rice
	
	Net Carbs: 22.6g; FV: 4g
		4–6 oz chicken
		1 small tomato
		2 cups mixed greens
		½ avocado
		2 Tbsp ranch dressing
		⅓ cup cooked lentils
		25 almonds
		Net Carbs: 18g; FV: 6.4g
			Atkins Frozen Beef
			  Merlot
			½ cup peas
			⅓ cup cooked sliced
			  carrots
			
			Net Carbs: 17.1g; FV: 4g
				4–6 oz ham or pork chop
				⅓ cup cooked lentils
				½ cup peas
				⅓ cup cooked sliced
				  carrots
				1 cup baby spinach
				½ avocado
				1 Tbsp ranch dressing
				Net Carbs: 21.3g; FV: 2.8g

SNACK	Atkins Advantage Coconut
	  Almond Delight Bar
	½ medium pear
	Net Carbs: 14g; FV: 0g
		½ medium apple
		1 oz Cheddar cheese
		
		Net Carbs: 8.9g; FV: 0g
			Atkins Advantage Café
			  Caramel Shake
			25 almonds
			Net Carbs: 4.8g; FV: 0g
				1 small tomato
				5 whole wheat crackers
				1 oz Cheddar cheese
				Net Carbs: 16.4g; FV: 2.5g

DINNER	4–6 oz canned tuna or
	  fish filet
	2 cups mixed greens
	½ avocado
	⅓ cup garbanzo beans
	2 Tbsp vinaigrette
	1 cup broccoli florets
	Net Carbs: 16.8g; FV: 5.6g
		Atkins Frozen Meatloaf
		  with Portobello
		  Mushroom Gravy
		¼ cup peas
		¼ cup brown rice
		
		Net Carbs: 21.1g; FV: 4g
			4–6 oz chicken
			1 cup broccoli florets
			2 cups mixed greens
			2 Tbsp creamy Italian
			  dressing
			½ medium pear
			
			Net Carbs: 15.5g; FV: 4.3g
				Atkins Frozen Chicken and
				Broccoli Alfredo
				½ cup cantaloupe cubes
				½ cup Greek yogurt
				
				Net Carbs: 15.6g; FV: 5g

	Total Net Carbs: 71.1g
	Total Net Carbs from
	  FV: 17.1g
		Total Net Carbs: 69.3g
		Total Net Carbs from
		  FV: 15.8g
			Total Net Carbs: 71.5g
			Total Net Carbs from
			  FV: 12.1g
				Total Net Carbs: 69.4g
				Total Net Carbs from
				  FV: 15.6g

Enjoy Atkins Endulge Treats for dessert if Net Carb consumption allows!

Friday	Saturday	Sunday
1 cup baby spinach	Atkins Frozen Tex-Mex	2 eggs
1 small tomato	Scramble	2 cups baby spinach
½ avocado	½ medium apple	1 tsp olive oil
1 oz Monterey Jack cheese	½ cup Greek yogurt	½ bell pepper
10 almonds		1 oz Monterey Jack cheese
½ cup tomato juice		½ cup cantaloupe cubes
Net Carbs: 10.8g; FV: 9.7g	**Net Carbs: 18.2g; FV:3g**	**Net Carbs: 12g; FV: 5.3g**
½ medium apple	Atkins Advantage Caramel	2 stalks celery
20 almonds	Chocolate Nut Roll	2 oz Cheddar cheese
	Bar	½ cup tomato juice
Net Carbs: 10.8g; FV: 2.5g	**Net Carbs: 3g; FV: 0g**	**Net Carbs: 7.1g; FV: 6.4g**
Atkins Frozen Roast	4–6 oz canned tuna or	Atkins Advantage
Turkey Tenders with	fish filet	Chocolate Peanut
Herb Pan Gravy	2 Tbsp mayonnaise or	Butter Bar
⅓ cup brown rice	tartar sauce	20 walnut halves
	2 stalks celery	½ medium pear
	¼ cup chopped bell pepper	
	1 small tomato	
	4 whole wheat crackers	
Net Carbs: 20g; FV: 4g	**Net Carbs: 16.9g; FV: 5g**	**Net Carbs: 15.8g; FV: 0g**
Atkins Advantage Caramel	Atkins Advantage Vanilla	1 cup sliced bell pepper
Chocolate Peanut	Shake	¼ cup hummus
Nougat Bar	25 almonds	
10 large strawberries	½ medium pear	
Net Carbs: 13.2g; FV: 0g	**Net Carbs: 14.8g; FV: 0g**	**Net Carbs: 8.7g; FV: 3.7g**
4–6 oz ham or pork chop	4 oz steak or hamburger	Atkins Frozen Crustless
1 cup broccoli	1 small tomato	Chicken Pot Pie
1 cup mixed greens	½ avocado	½ cup peas
⅓ cup garbanzo beans	½ small onion, sliced	*⅓ cup brown rice*
2 Tbsp creamy Italian	½ baked sweet potato	
dressing		
10 walnut halves		
Net Carbs: 15.4g; FV: 2.9g	**Net Carbs: 16.3g; FV: 6.4g**	**Net Carbs: 26.1g; FV: 4g**
Total Net Carbs: 70.3g	**Total Net Carbs: 69.2g**	**Total Net Carbs: 69.7g**
Total Net Carbs from	**Total Net Carbs from**	**Total Net Carbs from**
FV: 14.7g	**FV: 14.4g**	**FV: 19.4g**

PDQ SNACKS FOR PHASE 3 AND BEYOND

Your snack options expand in Pre-Maintenance (Fine-Tuning), although you can continue to enjoy tasty, convenient Atkins snacks and shakes. If you have the fixings in the fridge and pantry, you can also put together these tasty and portable snacks in minutes.

- Cottage cheese and orange slices
- Apple slices spread with almond or peanut butter
- Half a pear with blue cheese
- Greek yogurt with papaya slices
- Atkins Trail Mix: nuts, seeds, no-sugar-added shredded coconut, and a cut-up Atkins bar
- Prosciutto-wrapped pineapple
- Provolone-wrapped kiwi slices
- Carrot sticks with hummus
- Air-popped popcorn sprinkled with grated Parmesan cheese

EXERCISE: NO MORE EXCUSES

Okay, here I go again. Now that you're homing in on your goal weight, there's really no excuse not to add physical activity to your weight-control program. It might speed the loss of those last few pounds, and without question it will help you maintain your soon-to-be-achieved new weight. If you've started exercising regularly, you're already on the right track. And if you've been working out all along, it might be time to intensify your efforts.

The Centers for Disease Control recommend that adults get a minimum of two and a half hours of moderate-intensity exercise a week. But any physical activity is better than none, and if you're new to exercise, you can certainly begin with less and gradually increase in intensity and duration. Make sure to include both resistance exercise, also known as strength training, to increase your muscle endurance and strength, and cardiovascular exercise. You can achieve the former with hand weights or resistance bands, or simply by using your body weight, as you do with push-ups. Brisk walking, jogging, swimming, and bicycling are all great ways to achieve cardiovascular or aerobic exercise. Numerous websites offer videos and guided instruction.

WHAT TO EXPECT

The closer you get to your goal weight, the more your body resists letting go of its excess baggage. Take the following into consideration:

- *You may want to adjust your goal.* If you feel good about yourself at the weight you've achieved, terrific. You may have reached your natural weight, which is the one you can maintain easily. Or perhaps your original goal was too modest and you've realized that you could actually shave off even more pounds now that you've experienced such success on Atkins. If so, there's no reason not to dial your goal weight down another 10 pounds or so.
- *Take a break.* Or you may decide to hang out at a certain weight for a few months, get comfortable with it, and then take off the final 10 pounds.
- *It's not just about pounds.* Another possibility is that although your weight is a bit higher than you'd originally aimed for, you've lost inches and can fit into clothes you haven't worn in years. The point is that there is no magic number, just the right one for you.
- *You'll need to experiment to find your limits.* Figuring out which food you can or cannot handle is important for long-term weight control. Wouldn't you rather know for a fact that eating potatoes or bananas just isn't worth the price?
- *Your weight loss may slow to a crawl,* perhaps only a half pound a week. This is both deliberate—so that you can expand your carb

intake and food choices—and natural. Weight loss obviously slows the closer you get to where your body naturally "wants" to be. And losing slowly gives you time to get really comfortable as you transition to a permanent way of eating.

TROUBLESHOOTING

Even though you're almost at your goal, adding carbs and new foods can cause some frustrations. Here's how to handle them—or accept them.

- *You may experience cravings and uncontrollable hunger* as you add back foods you have not eaten in some time. See page 131 for how to proceed.
- *You may wind up on a plateau.* If you've already experienced one or more plateaus in OWL, you know all about that exercise in delayed gratification. If you've been spared this frustrating experience to date, my advice is to first ascertain that it's truly a plateau, meaning you're doing everything correctly. If so, reduce your daily Net Carb intake by 10 grams and wait it out as patiently as you can. For a review, see page 140.
- *You may stumble upon your Net Carb tolerance for weight maintenance* in what initially appears to be a plateau. To see if this is the case, step down 10 grams of Net Carbs daily for at least a week. If weight loss resumes, go up another 5 grams, and so forth.

MISSION ACCOMPLISHED? NOT QUITE

The day you've dreamed of for months has finally arrived. You've reached your goal weight! Whether you've melted away 20 pounds, shed 50 pounds, or joined the bye-bye-100-pounds club, congratulations on a job well done. Can you sit back and relax? Sure. Can you pat yourself on the back? Absolutely. Can you celebrate by pigging out on all those foods you've forsaken for the duration? No way! In fact, you aren't even ready to leave Phase 3 yet. How come? As the old saying goes, *losing* weight is easy; the hard part is *maintaining* your new weight. That's exactly what you begin to do in Phase 3, and that's why this phase is considered a dress rehearsal for Phase 4, Lifetime Maintenance. For the next four weeks your job is to maintain your goal weight.

PRACTICE MAKES PERFECT

To stay at your new weight, you need to know exactly how many grams of Net Carbs you can eat each day. Hint: it's usually 5 or 10 grams higher than the highest personal carb balance number you achieved while still losing weight. You'll also be assessing the ease or difficulty of keeping your weight constant at that level. The highest level of carb intake you can push yourself to may not be the level at which you're the most comfortable.

In addition to monitoring your weight for the next month, stay alert to those old familiar indicators that you know all too well from when you began Atkins: low energy, carb cravings, and unreasonable hunger. If you're dragging around, feeling jittery, lusting after certain foods, or ravenous by the time your next meal or snack rolls around, chances are you've pushed yourself too high. It's likely you're also having a hard time maintaining your new weight at this unsustainable level, although a swing of 2 or 3 pounds from day to day is normal. Continue to use weight averaging instead of a single day's weight as an indicator.

If you're struggling to maintain your weight at this level, simply back down by 5 grams of Net Carbs daily and see if that's easier to handle. If that doesn't do the job, go down another 5 grams. This process may involve some trial and error, during which you may also find that you've reintroduced certain foods that are giving you problems, perhaps by stimulating cravings or uncontrollable hunger. If you suspect that particular foods are sabotaging your progress, eliminate them for several days to see whether things improve before trying to introduce them again.

Once you find the number of grams of Net Carbs that's sustainable in terms of weight maintenance and the other indicators discussed above, remain at that level for four weeks before moving to Phase 4. Just to be clear, don't leave Phase 3 until your weight has remained constant for four weeks! This back-and-forth business may seem like a drag now that you've reached your goal weight. But knowing exactly what you can and cannot handle enables you to stay in control in the coming months—and years.

FREQUENTLY ASKED QUESTIONS

Q. How do I know when I've reached the right weight for me?
A. There is no single right or wrong weight. Your body type, age, hormonal status, activity level, and genetics all play a role. As we've discussed, you may be able to achieve a lower weight, but if it's a struggle to maintain it, you may want to accept that being 5 or even 10 pounds heavier is where your body naturally wants to be. Again, inches count as much as pounds. As you tone your abdominals and other muscles with regular physical activity, your body will appear slimmer. When you come to a point where you're comfortable with your weight at this time in your life, that's the place to remain.

Q. Can I eat any low-carb product when I'm in Phase 3?
A. In Phase 1, you can have low-carb foods with Net Carb counts of 3 grams per serving; that increases to 6 grams per serving in OWL, and to 9 grams in this phase. In Lifetime Maintenance, the number rises to 10 grams or more, assuming your carb tolerance allows.

Q. Can I have more than one or two glasses of wine now that I have reached my goal weight?

A. Yes, if it doesn't cause weight gain or leave you vulnerable to over-eating the snack foods that often accompany alcohol. I generally recommend a single glass for women and up to two for men, but you know your own tolerance. If you regain weight or lose control, drop back to a single glass or none. Also continue to avoid high-carb beer and mixers made with added sugar.

Q. Why am I experiencing cravings I haven't had for months?

A. There are two possible explanations. Either you're simply eating too many carbs and not burning primarily fat for energy anymore (remember, fat burning suppresses your appetite) or you've reintroduced a food or food group that's spiking your blood sugar. Fruit may be the culprit, particularly if you're not accompanying it with fat or protein to moderate the impact on your blood sugar. Cut back by 10 grams of Net Carbs a day and eliminate the foods you're added recently. Then reintroduce them slowly, one by one, to find out which ones are creating cravings.

Q. How can I tame my sweet tooth?

A. There are two approaches: satisfy it or eliminate it. Satisfy your sweet tooth with acceptable substitutes, such as an Atkins Endulge bar. If you're able to have such treats without overdoing them and without causing cravings, fine. If not, eliminate any foods that may be triggering cravings for sweets until you get the situation under control.

Q. What desserts can I have in this phase?

A. In addition to Endulge bars, plus the berries, cherries, and melon you started to eat in Phase 2, you can have almost any other fruit, as well as other desserts with no added sugar and no more than 9 grams of Net Carbs.

MOVING ON

The big question, of course, is how to know when to transition to Phase 4, Lifetime Maintenance. If you can answer all the following questions in the affirmative, go ahead. Otherwise, hold off until you have three yeses.

- Are you at your goal or adjusted goal weight?
- Has your weight remained constant for the last four weeks?
- Are cravings and undue hunger no longer a problem?

Before you get to Chapter 8, where you'll learn how to transition from a weight-loss program to a weight-maintenance program—that means the rest of your slim, energized, healthy life!—meet Gretchen M. Her ongoing weight-loss journey on Atkins is nothing less than amazing. She has already lost an unbelievable 300 pounds and still has another 100 to go. When you read her story you'll be as convinced as I am that she'll reach her goal weight—and stay there! Gretchen knows for a fact that she will never fall back into her old life. "I've been through it all and nothing will make me go back to the bad old days," she declares.

HITTING BOTTOM BEFORE SEEING THE LIGHT

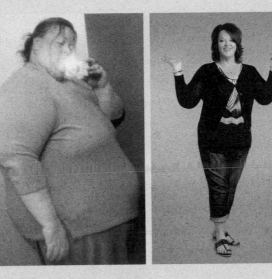

VITAL STATS

Daily Net Carb intake: 25–35 grams

Age: 37

Height: 6'1"

Before weight: 565 pounds (estimated)

After weight: 265 pounds

Lost: 300 pounds

Gretchen M. of Las Vegas has had it tough, starting with a childhood shaped by an alcoholic father and an abusive mother. Her marriage was not much better. Serious health problems, the loss of her career, and having to send her children away all caused the emotional distress that contributed to her obesity. But then Gretchen found Atkins. She's lost a remarkable amount of weight and knows the rest is just a matter of time. She credits

Atkins with helping her turn her life around. Gretchen shares her painful but ultimately transformative life story.

My doctor would never give me my starting weight because he thought it would demotivate me and no scale could hold me, so I'm not really sure how much I weighed at my heaviest. I needed instant gratification, so instead of setting a goal weight at the start I set mini goals, beginning with 5-pound losses; later, with every 10 pounds I lost I'd buy myself a charm for my weight-loss charm bracelet. I also took a picture of myself every three or four weeks in the same shirt after visiting my doctor and getting my current weight, and post both on my Facebook page.

Although I'm tall and I was always curvy, after I had my two children I could never get below 200 pounds. I was a nurse, but I crushed my knee and became addicted to painkillers, which ended that career. I then found a part-time job without benefits. Meanwhile, my husband and I divorced. Shortly afterward, I was diagnosed with cancer. The kids and I were living with my mother, but she couldn't handle the stress of my situation, so she kicked us out. Painful as this was, it was no surprise. When my father was dying of cancer years ago, my mother made me care for him. She beat me every day (and forbade me to cry) before I left home at fifteen.

I was unable to provide a decent place to live while I was undergoing chemo and radiation, so I signed over custody of my son and daughter to my ex's parents. They lived in Idaho, so I rarely saw the kids. One bright spot in this list of horrors was meeting my boyfriend six months before my cancer diagnosis. He has been by my side the whole time.

Over the Christmas holidays of 2010, I had my kids with me and we went shopping. I was so heavy I could barely walk and sweat was pouring off me. My son was taking forever to decide which shirt to get and mouthed off at me. I completely lost it and screamed at him. Everyone stared at us and I could tell by the look on both kids' faces that they were ashamed of me. It just tore me apart. After they left to go back to Idaho, I was this close to killing myself. Instead, I got up at five o'clock the next morning, went online, and found Atkins.

When I read about carbohydrates it was as though a light-bulb went off in my head. I've since changed my entire way of eating. Now if God made it, I eat it, meaning no sugar and no processed foods. When I eat out I know which questions to ask and what to order, but I prefer my own food because I know exactly what's in it.

I'm in Phase 2 now and my goal is to get to 160 pounds, which means losing another 105 pounds. I've already lost almost three times that, so I know I can do it. I'm very active, walking my dog like twelve times a day and working out regularly on a stationary bike.

I've survived an abusive childhood, a horrible marriage, destroying my knee, and losing my career, but now I know there's nothing I can't accomplish. Sometimes I have bad days, but now I can handle what once would have triggered a binge. As long as I follow Atkins, I can stay in control. I don't have to fill myself up to feel good. My brain is the calmest it has ever been. I don't understand it, but I live it!

I used to wear size 7X or 8X clothing, and even that was skintight on me. As I lost weight, I began to sell my fat-lady clothes on eBay. Then I branched out, finding other large-size items, and now have a thriving e-business. This new career has opened up a whole new world for me. More important, my cancer is in remission, my sixteen-year-old daughter is back home, and my son's in college, heading for law school. And when I look at my kids all I see is pride, not embarrassment, in their eyes.

MAKE IT EASY

I cook one day a week and freeze meals so I always have something I can pop in the microwave. One of my favorite snacks is whole-milk yogurt with peeled, sliced cucumbers. *—G.M.*

CHAPTER 8

WELCOME THE NEW YOU

You did it! You're finally in Phase 4, Lifetime Maintenance. You set a goal, made significant changes in your habits, stuck to your guns, and accomplished what you set out to do. You're probably receiving compliments left and right, along with looks of amazement from people who haven't seen you in a while. Exciting as all that attention can be, it's probably nothing compared to your own sense of pride and accomplishment. Pat yourself on the back and take a bow! And carve out time to celebrate your achievements, perhaps with some new formfitting clothes, a weekend at the beach, or a great new haircut and makeover. I also strongly recommend that you record your feelings about your weight-loss journey and the happy results in your journal. And don't forget to take an after photo of the svelte new you!

When you think about your accomplishments, don't stop with your streamlined body. If any of the following apply, congratulate yourself on them as well. For example, in the process of doing Atkins, did you do any of the following?

- Eliminate a destructive habit such as drinking sugary sodas, eating in front of the television, or having a daily doughnut at break time

- Develop a healthy new habit of a daily brisk walk or riding your bike to work, or start an exercise program or build upon an existing one
- Create weekly meal plans and shopping lists
- Develop a love of vegetables
- Improve your family's nutrition and sit down together for meals more often
- Honor your commitments to yourself
- Make other significant and positive changes in your life

THE LONG HAUL

In your current cloud of optimism you may be saying to yourself, "I've lost the weight and kept it off for a month, so what's the point of yet another phase of Atkins?" Whoa! That kind of thinking can set you up for a fall. Again, the last four weeks of Pre-Maintenance were only a rehearsal for Lifetime Maintenance, which is not so much a phase as a permanent lifestyle. Sad to say, this is where all too many people, regardless of how they lost weight, get cocky and soon find themselves in trouble. In fact, up to 95 percent of people who shed extra pounds on any weight-loss program regain it when they return to their old eating habits. Or they fall off the wagon and can't figure out how to climb back on. According to the National Weight Control Registry, people who keep off their lost pounds have several traits in common. They:

- Eat breakfast
- Exercise almost every day
- Monitor their weight regularly
- Track their food intake

The good news is that if you're following the Atkins program and you've opted to make physical fitness part of your life, there's no reason why you have to become part of that 95 percent. In many additional ways, Atkins is designed to make maintaining your weight easy. Here's why:

- You've transitioned from phase to phase, gradually increasing your carb intake, as you worked toward a permanent way of eating.
- By reintroducing foods one by one, you know which, if any, could spell trouble for you.
- You now know which foods you can do without and which you love but must eat in moderation.
- You've learned how to be alert to the signals of cravings or undue hunger and how to respond before you lose control.
- You've discovered how to substitute certain low-carb foods for high-carb ones, treat other foods as garnishes, and more.
- Most important, you've come to trust the Atkins program and experience the pleasure of feeling good, both physically and emotionally.

If you accept that Phase 4 is a lifestyle and act accordingly, I can promise that you'll never have to "diet" again. Does that mean that you won't ever regain a few pounds? Of course not. If you go on vacation and dine out every night, you may well pack on some excess baggage. If an injury lays you up for a few weeks and you can't get to your exercise class, some excess pounds may creep back. But now you possess the tools and skills, the same ones you've honed for months, to turn around any such situation. Just as important, don't succumb to negative thinking by letting an occasional misstep become a reason to wallow in guilt and punish yourself by falling into a downward spiral.

ACCEPTABLE PHASE 4 FOODS

In general, the foods you can eat in Lifetime Maintenance are the same ones you've already been eating, although you can now introduce

Atkins Cuisine Penne Pasta. There may be some foods you tried to reintroduce earlier without success that you can now handle. Feel free to experiment at any time as long as your weight remains under control. Just as there's great variation in how many carbs people can consume while losing weight, the same applies to weight maintenance. You might not be able to get much beyond 50 or 55 grams of Net Carbs a day (or even less), or you might be humming along at close to 100 grams or more.

FOOLPROOF ADVICE ON WEIGHT MAINTENANCE

To remain in control of your hard-won new weight:

- Stay at your carb tolerance level, the number of daily grams of Net Carbs you can consume while maintaining your weight. This is the threshold you discovered when you maintained your weight for a month in Phase 3 (Fine-Tuning).
- Continue to have a minimum of 12–15 grams of Net Carbs in the form of foundation vegetables.
- Continue to have 4–6 ounces of (cooked) protein at each meal.
- Aim for no more than two servings of fruit a day.
- Continue to see fat as your friend and integral to weight management.
- Combine carbohydrate foods with fat and/or protein to moderate your blood sugar response.
- Continue to drink plenty of water and other noncaloric beverages.
- Adjust your carb intake if you become less (or more) active.
- Distinguish between hunger and habit.
- Continue to weigh and measure yourself once a week.
- Never let yourself gain more than 5 pounds (unless you become pregnant) without taking immediate action.

- Add new foods one at a time to gauge their impact on cravings and appetite.
- Engage in regular physical activity.
- Portion out ahead of time any foods, such as nuts or cheese, that you might be tempted to overeat.
- Keep reading labels, especially on any new foods.
- Stay alert to the possibility of carb creep.
- Plan ahead if you decide to take an occasional departure from your low-carb lifestyle. (See "Taking a Break," page 186.)

APPETITE ADJUSTMENT

Now that you're maintaining rather than losing weight, you'll be consuming a slightly larger (with the emphasis on *slightly*) quantity of food, meaning more daily calories. Your appetite will also increase slightly at this point. As long as you're close to the weight your body "wants" to be, this is likely to occur naturally. Does that mean you'll also be consuming more carbs than you were in the last month of Pre-Maintenance? Not necessarily. You might be able, for example, to add a ½-cup serving of brown rice (about 21 grams of Net Carbs and about 108 calories) without experiencing cravings or undue hunger. In that case, you'd likely need to reduce your fat intake slightly.

On the other hand, if you have a lower carb tolerance, you'll have to make up that extra calorie demand with a bit more fat, perhaps with half a Hass avocado (less than 2 grams of Net Carbs and 153 calories) or 1 tablespoon almond butter (2.8 grams of Net Carbs and 102 calories). Unless you're eating less than 4 to 6 ounces of (cooked) protein at each meal, don't increase protein to boost calories. You may have to play a little with this adjustment so as to not overshoot the mark and start gaining weight. Continuing to make entries in your food journal should help you figure out which foods help fill you up without stimulating your appetite unnecessarily.

THE SCOOP ON SUGAR: STARTLING STATS

Toss these statistics from the USDA, Centers for Disease Control, and National Health and Nutrition Examination Survey around the next time someone asks why you've eliminated sugar from your diet.

- Each American consumes an average of 5 ounces of added sugars a day. That adds up to 116 pounds a year. If you're a woman, that might be your goal weight!
- We now consume more than twice as much fructose (fruit sugar), much of it in the form of high-fructose corn syrup, than we did thirty years ago.
- It's estimated that half of Americans drink one sweetened soda a day, and 5 percent have four or more—yes, in one day!
- On average, Americans eat a total of 30 teaspoons a day of added sugar in one form or another.
- The American Heart Association calls for an upper limit of 200 calories a day from added sugars. Which is more astounding, that a major health organization is this permissive or that most Americans consume far more than this amount?

NO WAY BACK

Here's a question I often hear from Atkins followers: "Now that I've lost weight, why can't I go back to my old way of eating but just be more moderate?" You're welcome to try, but I have to warn you that it's unlikely to work. You've learned that controlling your carb intake makes your body burn primarily fat for energy, which produces that wonderful side effect of moderating your appetite. Return to your old way of eating, and you'll be right back on the blood sugar roller coaster, experiencing peaks and dips in your energy level, which leads to overeating. Once more, Lifetime Maintenance is just that—a way of eating that you can sustain and which will maintain your healthy weight. The price you have to pay is small: continue to abstain from added sugar and refined grains, as well as anything that acts as a trigger food. Fortunately, there are so many tasty alternatives that this really isn't difficult, as we'll discuss in the next chapter.

AS TIME GOES BY

Perhaps you're in your forties or older and until recently never had to worry about your weight. Or perhaps you're in your twenties or thirties and assume that now you've slimmed down, you have it made. But things change, and your metabolism may be one of those things. That's why it's a good idea to understand that at some future date you may need to adjust your carb intake up or down in order to continue to maintain your weight. This may result simply from the passage of years, but here are a few other possible reasons to recalibrate:

- You may need to dial your daily Net Carb count down if:
  - ▶ An injury sidelines you for a few months.
  - ▶ A change in career puts you behind a desk eight hours a day.
  - ▶ You're prescribed a drug that slows your metabolism.
  - ▶ You enter menopause.

- You may need to dial your daily Net Carb count up if:
  - ▶ You take up a vigorous sport such as running or tennis.
  - ▶ You move to a fourth-floor walk-up apartment.
  - ▶ You're chasing after a toddler all day long.

Another very real possibility if you're a young woman is that you'll become pregnant. In this happy event, it's perfectly okay to continue with the Lifetime Maintenance phase of Atkins. See page 18 for more detail.

TAKING A BREAK

You may find yourself occasionally in a situation where you need to back off a bit on your low-carb lifestyle for a week or so. Perhaps you're visiting your new in-laws or traveling to another country where you'll be a guest in a private home. In either case, it could be impolite to not eat much of what's put on your plate. Or maybe you're in a new job and have to spend a week in training at the corporate office with all eyes on you. The best way to deal with such a situation is to plan ahead, perhaps by cutting down on your carbs for a week or two before. Also, be sure not to use such a situation as an excuse to pig out on desserts and other problematic foods. Finally, get back in gear immediately upon your return. Some more tips:

- At buffets, comply with your Atkins lifestyle, passing up white bread, white rice, gravy made with flour, and other obviously high-carb foods.
- In lieu of juice at breakfast, ask if fruit is available.
- Go easy on alcohol, which can interfere with your food inhibitions.
- Share desserts, have a small bite only, or ask for fruit instead.
- Pack some nuts and/or Atkins bars to keep your appetite under control between meals.
- Don't bore people by talking about how you usually eat.

TROUBLESHOOTING IN PHASE 4

Say you've gained 4 pounds and want to deal with the situation before it gets any more serious. Simply pare roughly 10 grams of Net Carbs a day from your intake until you return to your goal weight. Give or take a couple of grams, here are some candidates for subtraction:

- ½ banana
- 1 cup watermelon balls
- ½ large grapefruit
- 2 carrots
- ½ baked potato
- ¾ cup beets
- ½ small sweet potato
- ½ cup cooked oatmeal
- ¼ cup brown rice
- 1 slice whole-grain bread
- Scant ½ cup lentils
- ¾ cup shelled edamame
- ⅓ cup chickpeas
- 1 cup plain whole-milk yogurt

FREQUENTLY ASKED QUESTIONS

We all want to believe that once we've turned over a new leaf, the book stays open to that page. Now that you've reached your goal weight, you surely intend to stay there. But planning to do something and actually doing it aren't always the same. Let's look at some questions that frequently come up at this point in the program.

Q. What if my carb tolerance never goes above 50 grams of Net Carbs a day?

A. There's tremendous variation in how many carbs individuals can consume and still maintain their weight. Men have more muscle mass and therefore typically a higher metabolism, as do younger people. Hormonal issues also play a role. If you're sedentary, it's worth starting to work out. If you already exercise, increase your level of intensity and/or frequency to see if you can raise your carb tolerance level.

Q. I've been maintaining my weight nicely for several months. Can I occasionally have some of my old faves without upsetting the apple-cart?

A. Of course you can have a slice of cake at your kid's birthday party, for example, but plan for such occurrences, if possible, by cutting back on carbs for a day or two beforehand. If you find yourself constantly pushing the limits, however, there's a good risk that your occasional foray into the world of Starbucks sweetened drinks or eating a bag of chips on the way home from the supermarket could become a habit. The real risk isn't regaining a pound so much as losing the appetite control that Atkins provides.

Q. I've found that I can eat some sugary foods without gaining weight. Can I keep eating them?

A. Your metabolism may allow you do so without regaining weight, but as you've read in earlier chapters, added sugar is empty of real nutrients and has been implicated in the rise of obesity and diabetes. Eating such foods also displaces the nutritious vegetables and other whole foods that are relatively low in carbs. Keep eating these foods and you may find yourself on a slippery slope.

Q. What should I do when I occasionally succumb to temptation and eat an inappropriate food?

A. First of all, don't beat yourself up and then use that as an excuse to pig out for the rest of the day. The next day, simply return to following Phase 4 at your appropriate level of carb intake.

Q. On a two-week vacation, I gained back almost 10 pounds eating all sorts of foods I know I shouldn't have. How do I get back on track ASAP?

A. Being off your own turf and eating out day after day can disrupt your usual routines. The moment you get home, drop down 20 grams of Net Carbs from your usual amount. If a week at this level doesn't do the trick, return to Phase 2 until you achieve your goal weight again.

Q. After six months of maintaining my new weight, I fell off the wagon. How do I repair the damage?

A. Stress at home or work, losing your job, ending a relationship, or countless other changes in your life could push you back into your old habits. First and foremost, don't beat yourself up. You know how to lose the weight and how fragile that loss is. Return to Phase 2 until you're in control of your cravings, then gradually transition through the phases until you achieve and maintain your goal weight.

CAN YOU REMAIN SLIM FOREVER?

That's a tough question, but one that must be asked. How can you beat the odds I mentioned in the beginning of this chapter? Take this quiz to get a handle on whether you're vulnerable to regaining those excess pounds.

1. Have you gained, lost, and regained weight in the past?   Yes ___ No ___

2. Were you in a hurry to lose weight so you could eat your old favorite foods?   Yes ___ No ___

3. Do you eat to soothe yourself when you're depressed or under stress?   Yes ___ No ___

4. Do you still crave sugary or starchy junk foods?   Yes ___ No ___

5. Do you live with someone who doesn't support your new way of eating?   Yes ___ No ___

6. Do you enjoy the foods you can eat on Atkins?   Yes ___ No ___

7. Have you transitioned through the four phases of Atkins?   Yes ___ No ___

8. Have you discarded habits, such as noshing
   in front of the TV, that contributed to
   your weight gain?   Yes___ No ___
9. Do you eat regular meals?   Yes ___ No ___
10. Have you established a physical
    fitness regimen?   Yes ___ No ___

If you answered yes to several of the first five questions, you could be heading for trouble. Ditto if you responded no to a few of the second five questions. This book has laid out a program that makes Atkins a sustainable way of eating. If your answers make you concerned that you may be vulnerable to regaining lost weight, review the book to renew your commitment to maintaining the new you.

This test is not meant to discourage you. Rather, I want to encourage you to make Atkins your lifestyle. In the next two chapters, we'll look at how to incorporate Atkins meals into your life whether you're at home or away, as well as explore lots of great new products that make it easier than ever to eliminate empty carbs from your meals.

Now meet Natalie L., who has done just that and gone from wearing a size 28 to a size 1 or even a 0! By changing her way of eating, she also was able to dodge her family history of diabetes.

ELEVEN YEARS AND GOING STRONG

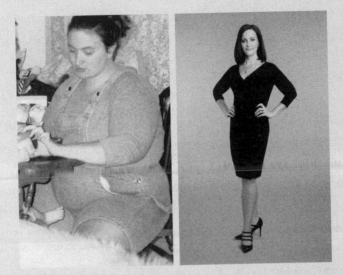

VITAL STATS

Daily Net Carb intake: 60 grams

Age: 37

Height: 5'6"

Before weight: 380 pounds

After weight: 120 pounds

Lost: 260 pounds

Like all too many women, Natalie L. had been overweight since she was a teenager and had tried multiple weight-loss programs without success. And like many other mothers, her pregnancies had aggravated the problem. Being at risk for diabetes didn't help either. But all that was more than a decade ago. Today, the Grayson, Georgia, resident is full of health and energy and is less than one-third of her pre-Atkins weight. Natalie fills in the details.

Diabetes runs in my family, and I was diagnosed as prediabetic when I was seventeen. I was told to avoid sugar and other high-carb foods, but I resisted that advice. After all, my favorite foods were ice cream and fried anything. In my family a vegetable was a french fry! Both my parents are overweight and take loads of medications. When we were growing up I was always the funny, chubby one and my sister was the thin, pretty one.

In 2002, when my second son was about eight months old, I knew I had to make a change. I was desperate to finally find something that worked so that I could feel better and keep up with both my babies. I found an Atkins book in a used-book store and figured I had nothing to lose but the fat. I felt terrible for the first two weeks. Now I realize I was not getting enough salt. I'd grown up on southern cooking, washing down deep-fried food with Diet Coke! But soon I felt amazing.

My husband had said that we could have another baby if I lost 100 pounds, which was a big motivator. It took me about nine months to reach that goal, and I got pregnant shortly thereafter. I talked to my doctor about staying on Atkins during the pregnancy and he said that was fine as long as I moved beyond Induction and ate more vegetables. He was much happier with my being 100 pounds lighter and doing Atkins than eating double cheeseburgers and french fries, as I had with the last two pregnancies. This time I gained only 8 pounds, and a day after the birth of my third son, I weighed less than I did before I'd become pregnant.

I went back to Induction afterward to lose the rest of the weight. Its strictness gave me the self-control I needed. I now wear a size 0 or 1, a major change from my old size 28! Until I lost the weight I'd never realized that I had a small frame. Today my blood sugar and blood pressure are normal, as is my cholesterol. Four years after I'd lost the weight, I was diagnosed with celiac disease. It was far easier for me than it is for most people to avoid foods with gluten in them because I was already living the Atkins lifestyle.

The control thing was huge for me. Having two babies within 21 months of each other meant that my life was all about everyone else. Atkins lets me take control of my body and my life. When I got married I was only twenty. My now ex-husband is a police officer and he used to control what we ate, when we went to the grocery store, and even what I wore. He wasn't happy with the new independent me and didn't like all the attention I was getting. And losing weight made me realize that everything that was wrong with our marriage wasn't my fault. We divorced three years ago and I remarried a year later. My new husband eats the way I do with one exception: no way is he giving up his beer!

We're both very active. He plays tennis and I work out every single day. I joined a twenty-four-hour gym about a month after I started Atkins. I would go after the kids were in bed so that no one would see my fat butt! I started walking on a treadmill and later switched to a better gym, and now I have a gym in the house. I find I do best at about 60 grams of Net Carbs a day. If I go any higher, my skin breaks out and I get headaches. I still have a carb counter on my phone. My weight varies within a 5-pound range and I can dial it down if necessary.

Today I'm a Realtor and executive assistant, a job I never could have gotten when I was obese. It's still hard to see people who can eat everything, but nothing tastes good enough to be worth becoming the "fat girl" again. Now I know that I will live to see my boys grow up.

MAKE IT EASY

When we go on vacation, I take a tape measure to make sure I'm "behaving" in case I can't weigh myself. —*N.L.*

PART III

IT'S ALL ABOUT FOOD

CHAPTER 9

IT'S EASY TO EAT AT HOME

Which statement best describes you?

- I love to cook.
- I hate to cook.
- I have no time to cook.
- I cook occasionally.
- I do my real cooking on the weekends.

Or are you a combination of several of the above, depending upon your mood, day, workload, and other commitments? If you're like me, you may enjoy cooking when entertaining friends and family but not the pressure to cook every night. Or perhaps you're worried that making food suitable for Atkins is more complicated than "regular" cooking. (If someone else does most of the cooking in your family, share this chapter with him or her.)

Regardless of your attitude toward cooking, I can assure you that it's perfectly possible to get tasty, low-carb meals suitable for the whole family on the table with a minimum of time and fuss. Whether you're looking for quick and easy recipes, no-cook meals, make-in-advance meals, cook-while-you're-away meals, or cook-once-and-eat-twice meals, you'll find multiple solutions to the eternal problem of what to have for dinner tonight. Similar options apply to breakfast and lunch. Recipes begin on page 245 and are coded to indicate whether they contain a minimal number of ingredients, have a prep time of twenty minutes or less, are do-ahead meals, or can be made in a slow cooker.

MEALS FOR THE WHOLE FAMILY

Let's dispel one myth. There's no need to cook two separate meals, one for you and another for the rest of the family. Likewise, if you live alone, you can serve visitors the same foods you're eating without occasioning any strange looks. That's because Atkins-style cooking isn't that different from "regular" cooking. The key difference is the avoidance of certain ingredients, such as sugar, refined grains, and vegetable oil, and of breading and deep-frying food.

Basically, you simply subtract (or substitute) one or more items from the menu that the rest of the family will be eating. Here are some examples of how to feed the family while complying with your own needs with a minimum of extra work. And when a family meal is really high in carbs, Atkins products, including the frozen meals, can be a lifesaver.

THEM	YOU
Scrambled eggs and bacon with toast	Scrambled eggs and bacon with sliced tomatoes
Hot dogs on rolls, baked beans, cucumber spears	Hot dogs, sauerkraut, cucumber spears
Roast chicken, steamed spinach, baked sweet potatoes	Roast chicken, steamed spinach, celery spears with blue cheese dressing
Cereal with blueberries and milk	An Atkins Advantage bar and blueberries*
Beef burger on a bun; side salad, steamed green beans, french fries	Beef burger; side salad, steamed green beans

* In Phase 2

ALL IN THE FAMILY

Dinner is the most likely time that the family eats together. Your decision to go on Atkins may throw a curveball into family dynamics at first, until it becomes clear that Atkins is simply a healthy way to eat. Some advice:

- *If you're the primary cook:* Assure your partner that his or her meal preferences will be honored. For example, if pasta or another starchy dish is a must in your partner's book, you might make grilled salmon, a salad, and pasta for dinner and simply pass on the pasta. And really, how much trouble is it to boil the water for pasta, pop some potatoes in the oven, or steam rice in a microwave packet? If it preserves domestic harmony as you lose weight, why not?
- *If your mate is the chef:* Explain that there's not going to be any extra work. Any meal is fine as long as there is a protein source such as chicken or burgers without a starchy sauce, plus a vegetable and/or salad. If mac and cheese or another high-carb meal is on the menu, simply pop an Atkins frozen meal in the microwave for yourself. Or swap out vegetables in a starchy sauce with a salad from a salad bar.

FAMILY POLITICS

Changing the way you eat can make your nearest and dearest uncomfortable. A conversation with your partner and/or kids can usually eliminate any concerns. And then there's the matter of your extended family. Let's take these one by one.

- *Significant others.* If you're lucky, your partner understands your reasons for deciding to lose weight and respects your choice of Atkins. She or he may even be joining you on the program. On the other hand, your main squeeze might feel threatened by your decision, particularly if she or he is also overweight. Or your partner may simply not understand how cutting carbs and eating healthy fats can result in dramatic weight loss. If so, suggest reading Chapter 1 of this book. Make sure not to disparage his or her weight or knowledge of nutrition. Also make it clear that you're not asking permission to do Atkins. Simply explain that you believe this is right for you and you'd appreciate understanding.

- *Kids.* If parents are relaxed and comfortable with the offerings at mealtime, the fact that you're doing Atkins should be a nonissue. Obviously younger kids will react, if at all, differently than teens. Assure kids that family meals won't change; you just may not eat everything they eat. As long as the way you eat doesn't threaten them, kids should be fine. They might even follow your lead as they see you snacking on nuts and eating lots of veggies and simply prepared protein dishes. Never nag your children about eating too much of something or not enough of another food, and never bring up their weight in the context of a meal.

- *Extended family.* Eating habits can carry a lot of emotional freight in some families. Your sister, mother, mother-in-law, or grandmother could feel threatened by your decision to start on Atkins, especially if she is also overweight. In cultures with strong culinary traditions, your new way of eating, sans pasta or tortillas, for example, could make your relatives feel you're rejecting family traditions. Reassure them that you're not impugning their apple pie, calzones, beef burritos, or Yorkshire pudding. Rather, losing weight is something you need to do to feel good about yourself. Explain that that's why you won't be eating a particular food (even just a taste) at the next family dinner. Make it clear that you respect their choices and trust that they will respect yours. By all means, don't act superior (a risk for new converts of any sort) or challenge their culinary approach.

Now let's get down to how to make it easier to get food on the table. We'll cover the gamut from meals you can toss together from pantry staples and leftovers to main-dish salads, quick stir-fry and slow-cooker dishes, and more. Among these choices, you're sure to find some that suit your culinary preferences and cooking style.

NO-TIME-TO-SHOP MEALS

Your first objective is to always have Atkins-appropriate food available. You can find all the basics you'll need in a supermarket or warehouse club. If you cook regularly, you probably already have a number of those basics on hand. You don't necessarily have to have everything in the kitchen at all times. For example, if you shop weekly, you may not need more than one or two protein sources in the freezer. But once you fill your fridge, freezer, and pantry (and restock regularly) with acceptable foods, you'll never find yourself with "nothing to eat."

NO-COOK MEALS

Sometimes I'm just too bushed to make dinner after work, but the last thing I want to do is eat out. I'd much rather chill out at home in my sweats and slippers. I'm sure you often feel the same way. Of course, takeout is an option, but it's almost as pricey as eating at a restaurant. What to do?

Fortunately, with salad bars, delis, and a whole array of ready-to-serve products at the supermarket, you have another set of options. The granddaddy of such offerings is the rotisserie-roasted chicken. After a short pit stop, you'll be able to assemble a no-cook meal in minutes. A word of caution: many foods in delis and salad bars are full of high-carb ingredients, so ask questions, read labels, and avoid meats cured with nitrates or made with bread crumbs and other fillers, starchy sauces, and salads with added sugar.

From the Deli

- Rotisserie-roasted chicken; chicken, tuna, egg, whitefish, or shrimp salad; smoked salmon; grilled, roasted, poached, or broiled chicken; chopped liver
- Ham, pastrami, corned beef, salami,* brisket, roast or smoked turkey, grilled chicken breast
- Sauerkraut, pickles, pickled green beans, pickled mushrooms, cucumber salad, coleslaw

From the Salad Bar

- Grilled, roasted, or baked turkey, salmon, tuna, and chicken; grilled or steamed shrimp; tofu; hard-boiled eggs; deviled eggs
- Grilled, braised, or steamed broccoli, asparagus, cauliflower, green beans, and other foundation veggies (without problematic sauces)
- Salad greens, tomatoes, avocado, and other salad veggies
- Olives, hummus (in Phase 2), baba ganoush (eggplant dip)
- Berries and melon balls (in Phase 2); additional fruit (in Phase 3 or 4)
- Nuts, seeds, crumbled bacon, grated cheese
- Feta cheese, Cheddar cheese, etc.
- Vinaigrette, blue cheese, or ranch dressing
- *What to avoid:* meats and fish with starchy sauces, croutons, crunchy noodles, bean salads (unless you're in Phase 2), pasta salads, and other composed salads with off-limits ingredients; imitation crab (surimi); sushi; stuffed grape leaves; crackers.

From the Supermarket

In addition to the pantry staples listed above, check out:

- Bumble Bee fully cooked salmon fillets or albacore tuna steaks, which come in convenient 4-ounce portions

---

* Avoid products with nitrates

- Bagged coleslaw and washed and bagged salad mixes
- Trimmed and cut-up vegetables and fruits

Put It All Together
Here are a few no-cook combos for busy nights:

- Grilled chicken with green beans and salad from the salad bar
- A bagged salad topped with a tuna steak and asparagus
- Corned beef with sauerkraut and cucumber salad
- Smoked turkey over coleslaw with ranch dressing
- Sliced panino, sliced ham, and antipasto items such as marinated artichoke hearts, roasted bell peppers, mushrooms, olives, and feta cheese
- Grated zucchini topped with a salmon steak and pesto

WHEN A SALAD IS PLENTY

A robust salad can be the main attraction, rather than just an accompaniment to a meal. Plus, most salads can also be prepared in minutes. Our recipe developer has come up with five zingers, starting on page 270, all of which are suitable for all phases of Atkins:

- Chipotle Shrimp Salad
- Grilled Chicken and Marinated Kale Salad
- Buffalo Chicken Salad
- Turkey Enchilada Salad
- Crisp Lettuce Wedge with Sliced Flank Steak

You can also check atkins.com for more main dish salad recipes.

MEALS ON THE DOUBLE

Next up are meals you can prepare with minimal fuss and muss, thanks to a host of products ready to heat up in the microwave or on the cooktop. You'll find such time-savers as you prowl the grocery store, starting with our own Atkins frozen meals. This new line of comfort foods includes Beef Merlot, Meatloaf with Mushroom Gravy, and Crustless Chicken Pot Pie, all brimming with flavor but without the extra carbs and added sugar. (Go to atkins.com/products for a store locator.) Unfortunately, most other prepared foods often involve a trade-off between certain ingredients and convenience, so read food labels carefully.

- Skip the sea of fish sticks, fish cakes, and other battered or breaded prepared fish dishes and seek out the few acceptable alternatives, including grilled tilapia, salmon, and pollock. Gorton's Cajun Grilled Fillets (pollock) have no unacceptable ingredients, but the grilled salmon and tilapia dishes contain trace added sugars and starches. Some of Mrs. Paul's and Van de Kamp's baked and grilled fish dishes contain added sugar in marinades, which you can discard after cooking.
- You can also find several kinds of frozen fish fillets in individual-portion vacuum-sealed bags. Remove from the freezer in the morning to defrost in the fridge. Unbreaded frozen shrimp, scallops, and calamari also come in handy for quick stir-fries.
- Look for frozen tilapia, shrimp, and other fish entrées that cook in a marinade of lemon juice and other seasonings inside parchment cooking bags.
- Chicken tenders, individually packaged burgers, lamb or pork chops, and sausages are other good quick-cooking protein option. As with fish, pair with a cooked vegetable and a salad.

- Top grilled pork chops or meatballs with jarred marinara sauce. Or serve chicken, turkey breast, or veal with a jarred Alfredo sauce. Look for products without added sugar such as Amy's Family Marinara or Patsy's, Prego, or Walden Farms marinara sauces, as well as Bertolli Light, Di Giorno, and Walden Farms Alfredo sauces. (Not all products from these brands have no added sugar; read labels carefully.)

- Simmer sauces let you put together a curry in minutes. Simply heat leftover chicken or another meat, shrimp, or packaged chunks of grilled or roasted chicken or turkey in the sauce. Add some frozen veggies and serve over brown rice (or spaghetti squash, bean sprouts, or grated zucchini if you're not eating whole grains). Check out products by Trader Joe, Devya, and Simmering Secrets, among others, always staying on guard for added sugars.

- Frozen veggies in microwave steamer bags are a speedy option and eliminate having to wash another pot. Just be sure to purchase those without sauces made with starches and/or added sugar. You can also buy steamer bags and add your own mix of fresh or frozen veggies, including sauce or seasonings. Note that these bags *do not* contain BPA or phthalates.

MAKE IT EASY

To save on cleanup time, bake individual fish fillets or chicken tenders in a tightly sealed foil packet placed on a cookie sheet. Before sealing the packet, add a pat of butter, some thinly sliced vegetables, and seasonings. Bake in a 400°F oven for 20–25 minutes.

SAVE AS YOU SLIM DOWN

There are countless inexpensive low-carb options, and the first step to keeping a lid on costs is to plan your meals and recipes for the week.

Having meal makings at hand prevents you from having to make last-minute runs to the supermarket, hitting the drive-through, or ordering takeout for dinner. Here are more ways to start saving:

- *Choose cheaper cuts.* There's no need to eat pricey beef tenderloin. Sirloin and chuck contain more fat, making them flavorful, tender, juicy, and well suited to slow-cooking dishes such as stews, soups, and roasts. Lamb shanks, ham steaks, rib and shoulder pork chops, and pork, chicken, or turkey sausages are other budget-friendly choices. Buy meat in bulk when certain cuts are on sale and freeze in single or family-size portions.
- *Pass on chicken parts.* Whole chickens are almost always less expensive per pound than packaged parts. Cut them up or roast a whole bird for several meals over the course of a week.
- *Go fish.* Don't assume that salmon, flounder, shrimp, and scallops are the only way to go. Bluefish, catfish, tilapia, sardines, mackerel, and mussels are less pricey options.
- *Think beyond fish, poultry, and meat.* Eggs, legumes, and tofu and other soy foods can stand in for the usual protein sources. Ground turkey is another economical choice. Vegetarian protein crumbles or sausage can substitute for ground beef in chili and other recipes.
- *Bag the bag.* Washed, chopped, and bagged salad greens are a time saver but are always more expensive than head lettuce or other greens.
- *Shop in bulk.* If you don't already belong to a warehouse club, consider joining. Some supermarkets also now have bulk food sections where you can save on nuts, seeds, legumes, and whole grains.
- *Cheaper by the gallon.* Instead of purchasing bottled or canned soft drinks, make big batches of low-carb lemonade, iced tea, and coffee drinks, using an acceptable sweetener. Or flavor

water with a squeeze of lemon or lime or a few springs of mint. You'll be helping the planet while pinching pennies.

COOK ONCE, EAT TWICE

One way to save both time and dollars is to double or even triple recipes and freeze some, perhaps in individual portions for future meals. Or let a dish such as our Deep-Dish Sausage and Cauliflower Pizza (page 258) or Cheesy Chicken and Green Bean Skillet (page 259) do double duty as lunch the following day. Stews and slow-cooker dishes such as Crockpot Pork and Salsa Verde (page 262) are great candidates for doubling the recipe, as are soups such as Salmon Mushroom Chowder (page 283) and No-Bean Chicken Chili (page 279). You can also "remodel" leftover vegetables, for example, by adding broth and some leftover chicken or meat to make a hearty soup suitable for lunch on its own.

Experienced cooks know that for all its impressive presentation, making a roast beef, pork loin, chicken, or leg of lamb is easy to do—set the timer and forget about it. That weekend dish then pays dividends for the rest of the week. It's a time-honored way to get several meals out of one purchase and make the most of leftovers. A large roast chicken, for instance, could provide chicken salad for lunch the next day, chicken curry the following evening, and stir-fry with Asian veggies later in the week. If you're feeling industrious, you can even use the carcass to make chicken broth. Pretty good for an investment of about $12! The leftovers from beef, pork, and lamb roasts provide just as many opportunities for creativity. Once you open your mind to the possibilities, you'll learn to love leftovers.

SPEEDY STIR-FRIES

You don't need a wok to put together a tasty one-dish meal—a skillet will do the job. Technically, stir-frying takes place at a higher temperature than sautéing, but both techniques require cutting food up into small pieces and frequent turning and stirring to hasten the cooking process. Cutting up ingredients requires the most time, but you can take a shortcut by purchasing fresh vegetables already cut up. Most supermarkets offer them, or pick them up at a salad bar. Or use frozen veggies. Nor are Asian seasonings a must; try stir-fries that draw from other cuisines as well. A few possibilities:

- Asian Beef Stir-Fry (page 260)
- Cheesy Chicken and Green Bean Skillet (page 259)

From atkins.com:

- Spicy Orange Stir-Fry
- Beef, Scallions, and Red Bell Pepper Sauté
- Sautéed Scallops with Spinach Cream
- Snow Pea and Water Chestnut Stir-Fry*
- Stir-Fried Shrimp with Ginger and Mushrooms

You'll find that it's easy to modify the recipes in this book by swapping out one ingredient for another. So if a recipe calls for pork tenderloin, the same amount of chicken breast or sirloin can usually make a fine substitute. Likewise, if a recipe calls for asparagus and they're not in season or too expensive, green beans or broccoli can stand in.

* Add leftover chicken or pork to make a main dish.

A SLOW BUT STEADY SILENT HELPER

It may seem counterintuitive, but a slow cooker, aka crockpot, may be just what you need to get meals on the table *fast*. If you work outside the home or are ferrying your kids here, there, and everywhere, it almost allows you to be in two places at once. Slow cooking intensifies flavors and tenderizes meats, also making it ideal for cheaper cuts. In addition to delicious soups and stews, recipes for casseroles, curries, and roasts are easily adapted to the slow cooker. Here's a week's worth of easy recipes that lend themselves to this way of cooking.

- Crockpot Pork and Salsa Verde (page 262)
- No-Bean Chicken Chili (page 279)
- Salmon Mushroom Chowder (page 283)
- Taco Soup (page 280)

At atkins.com:

- Corned Beef and Cabbage
- Cranberry-Ginger Pork Roast
- Ropa Vieja

A SMARTPHONE IN THE KITCHEN

Once upon a time if you had a great meal at a restaurant you might rave about it on the phone to a friend the next day. Or if you turned out a particularly delish dish, you could share your excitement by scanning and sharing the recipe. But today you can snap a picture with your smartphone, boast about your success on countless websites, or simply text your mom or another good cook for advice on a recipe or an ingredient. Many mobile apps, including the app you can download at atkins.com, also make it easier to prepare meals by helping you make up a shopping list, "clip" coupons, compare prices, and plan meals—all in one place.

THE SCOOP ON SUGAR: SWEET AND SAVORY SUBSTITUTES

You expect to find added sugar in sweets, but it also all too often turns up in savory sauces and other products where you wouldn't expect it. Fortunately, many large food companies now manufacture sugar-free or no-sugar-added versions of their brands, including those listed below. Specialty companies have also stepped up to the plate with sugar-free versions of favorite foods. All of the following replacements are acceptable in Phase 1. Some, such as Heinz and Jell-O products, can be found in the supermarket. Others may need to be ordered online (see "Low-Carb Resources," on page 212, for URLs).

INSTEAD OF:	TRY THIS:
Starbucks flavored coffee drinks	Coffee plus Flavour Creations Tablets
Marshmallows	La Nouba Sugar-Free Marshmallows
Hard Candy	Life Savers Sugar Free
	Jolly Rancher Sugar Free
	Crystal Light
Twizzlers	Twizzlers Sugar Free
Barbecue sauce	Walden Farms Barbecue Sauce
	Trinity Hill Farms Barbecue Sauce
	Hallman's Bear Creek BBQ & Grilling Sauce
Heinz Ketchup	Heinz Reduced Sugar Ketchup
	Walden Farms Ketchup
A1 or Lea & Perrins Steak Sauce	Trinity Hill Steak Sauce
Hershey Chocolate Syrup	Hershey Sugar Free Chocolate Syrup
Del Monte Cocktail/Seafood Sauce	Walden Farms Seafood Sauce
Jell-O Pudding	Jell-O Sugar Free Pudding

SWAP THE SAUCE

Are you in a rut of serving the same five or six dishes week after week: "If it's Wednesday, it must be pork chops"? It's understandable that saving time is high on your list of priorities, but that needn't mean mealtime monotony. Easy-to-make sauces, marinades, and dressings can spice up plain fish, chicken, or meat dishes. Find several sauces you like and use them on a variety of protein choices. Add a vegetable and perhaps a side salad, and dinner can be on the table in minutes. Use the five sauces in the recipe section on a variety of protein sources and add a phase-appropriate vegetable or salad to each combo, and you won't have to repeat yourself for months. Plus you'll find almost two hundred more sauce-and-entrée combos in the Atkins recipe database.

SAUCE	PROTEIN SOURCE	SUITABLE SAUCES
1. Lemon Tartar	Chicken tenders	1, 2, 3, 4, 5
2. Chipotle BBQ Sauce	Pork chops	2, 3, 4, 5
3. Creamy Sweet Soy	Turkey sausages	2, 3, 4, 5
4. Red Wine Peppercorn	Skirt steak	2, 3, 4, 5
5. Fast Spicy Tomato	Hamburgers	1, 2, 4, 5
	Salmon	1, 2, 3, 4
	Shrimp	1, 2, 3, 4, 5
	Tilapia	1, 2, 3, 4, 5
	Ham steak	2, 3, 4
	Tofu cubes	2, 3, 4

CLASSICS, ATKINS STYLE

Foods such as mashed potatoes, fajitas, beef stroganoff, and french fries seem to be an integral part of our DNA! These classics are sky high in carbs and we know we shouldn't eat them—or at least only on special occasions—but they're darn near irresistible. Fortunately, there are ways to fool your taste buds with persuasive substitutes. Compare the comparable servings of a low-carb alternative to the classic dish to make your decision easy:

CLASSIC	ATKINS ALTERNATIVE	REDUCTION IN NET CARBS
Mashed potato	Mashed cauliflower	78%
French fries	Baked sweet potato "fries"	66%
French fries	Turnip fries	87%
Chili con carne	No-Bean Chicken Chili*	55%
Beef stroganoff on egg noodles	Beef stroganoff on shredded zucchini	90%
Beef stroganoff on egg noodles	Beef stroganoff on Atkins Cuisine Penne Pasta	53%
Deep-dish pizza	Deep-Dish Sausage and Cauliflower Pizza*	86%
Spaghetti and meatballs	Spaghetti squash and meatballs	90%

* Recipe included in this book.

LOW-CARB RESOURCES

You can, of course, order Atkins Advantage bars and shakes, Day Break bars, Endulge treats, and Atkins Cuisine All Purpose Baking Mix and Penne Pasta at atkins.com, as well as find them in retail outlets. The following companies manufacture or sell other Atkins-friendly foods you may want to explore. Some are available at supermarkets and discount clubs; others may need to be ordered online. Many sites have a store locator feature. This is hardly a complete list, but it should give you an idea of the range of low-carb products available.

- Asher's sugar-free candy, including toffee, caramel, and chocolate; ashers.com
- Better Bowls sugar-free gelatin and pudding mixes; betterbowls .com
- Big Train low-carb hot cocoa and other beverage mixes and cookie mixes; bigtrain.com
- Bob's Red Mill low-carb bread mix and almond, coconut, flax-seed, and hazelnut flour or meal; bobsredmill.com

- CarLO CARBiano low-carb pizza crusts, frozen pizzas, almond and flaxseed flour or meal, and breading mixes; carlocarbiano.com
- Cheesecake Factory no-sugar-added cheesecake; thecheese cakefactory.com
- Country Cupboard no-sugar-added fruit preserves, apple butter, and flavored syrup; countrycupboardinc.com
- DaVinci Gourmet sugar-free syrups and sauces; davincigour met.com
- Dixie Diners' Club low-carb and sugar-free products, including cake, muffin, cookie, and bread mixes, nut flours or meals, breakfast cereals, and Thick It Up gravy thickener; dixiediner .com
- Flavour Creations sugar free coffee flavoring tablets; flavour creations.com
- Genisoy low-carb soy chips, crisps, and soy nuts; genisoy.com
- Hallman's Bear Creek sugar-free BBQ sauces; hallmansbear creek.com
- Healthy Joy Bakes flaxseed bread with 1 gram Net Carbs per slice; healthyjoybakes.com
- Junior's no-sugar-added cheesecake; juniorscheesecake.com
- King's Cupboard sugar-free dark chocolate sauce and hot cocoa mix; kingscupboard.com
- Kitchen Table Bakers all-cheese crisps; kitchentablebakers.com
- Kozy Shack no-sugar-added puddings; kozyshack.com
- La Nouba sugar-free preserves, marshmallows, and a chocolate hazelnut spread that tastes like Nutella, all made in Belgium; lanouba.be
- LC Foods low-carb, sugar-free, gluten-free crackers, breads, frosting mixes, preserves, sweeteners, and thickeners; holdthe carbs.com
- MiRico low-carb breads, bagels, buns, and tortillas; mirico breads.com
- Rhythm Superfoods kale chips; rhythmsuperfoods.com

- Smucker's fruit jam, jelly and fruit preserves, dessert toppings, and syrups made without added sugar; smuckers.com/sensibly_sweet/product_list
- So Delicious almond, coconut, and soy milk unsweetened and sugar-free beverages, creamers, yogurt, and frozen desserts; sodeliciousdairyfree.com
- Steel's Gourmet Foods sugar-free sweeteners, syrups, and dessert sauces; steelsgourmet.com
- Trinity Hill Farms no-sugar-added sauces, salad dressings, and condiments; trinityhillfarms.com
- True Lemon no-carb citrus-flavored beverage mixes; truelemon.com
- Walden Farms no-sugar-added preserves, spreads, syrups, salad dressings; waldenfarms.com
- Wink dairy-free and no-sugar-added frozen desserts; winkfrozendesserts.com

THE SCOOP ON SUGAR: NATURAL, BUT STILL SUGAR

Mother Nature produces honey, maple syrup, molasses, and agave syrup, which all boast traces of antioxidants, but all of these still deliver a dense dose of carbs, as you can see below.

PRODUCT	AMOUNT	NET CARBS
Table sugar	1 tablespoon	12.6g
Agave nectar	1 ounce	20g
Honey	1 tablespoon	17g
Molasses	1 tablespoon	15g
Maple syrup	1 tablespoon	15g

BETTER CHOCOLATE CHOICES

Everyone loves chocolate, but most chocolate treats are sugar bombs. Instead, opt for substitutes for old favorites and you'll slash your sugar and carb intake. Put some of these products to the taste test.

HAVE THIS	INSTEAD OF THAT	QUANTITY	DIFFERENCE IN NET CARBS
Atkins Day Break Creamy Chocolate Shake	Chocolate Ice Cream Shake	11 oz	75g
Atkins Endulge Caramel Nut Chew	Snickers	1 bar	30g
Atkins Endulge Chocolate Caramel Mousse	Milky Way	1 bar	34g
Breyer's Carb Smart Chocolate Ice Cream	Breyer's Chocolate Ice Cream	½ cup	12g
Canfield's Diet Chocolate Fudge Soda	Yoo-Hoo	12 ounces	51g
La Nouba Chocolate Hazelnut Spread	Nutella	1 tablespoon	9g

FREQUENTLY ASKED QUESTIONS

Q. Do I have to rewash prewashed greens?
A. These veggies are a great convenience, but it's still a good idea to rinse and give them a whirl in a salad spinner. Greens usually stay crisp for up to five days when placed in a resealable plastic bag with a damp paper towel.

Q. I know I shouldn't eat them, but I still crave the crunch and saltiness of pretzels and chips. What do you recommend instead?
A. Actually, there are several alternatives. Rather than buying salted nuts or seeds, you could lightly sprinkle them with salt to moderate the inclination to keep eating them. Air-popped popcorn sprinkled

with Parmesan cheese or a bit of seasoned salt is fine in moderation in later phases of Atkins. Low-carb soy and veggie chips may also satisfy you. You can also find bagged kale chips, often flavored with grated cheese, which supply the crunch without the carbs. Finally, pork rinds are a fallback if you're still in the early phases of Atkins.

Q. Now that I'm maintaining my weight, can I have ice cream?

A. An occasional ½ cup of ice cream is not going to make you balloon up, but it may be hard to have just a small serving. A better approach is to explore ice creams made without added sugar, including some by Breyer's, Dreyer's, and Edy's. Other frozen low-carb treats include fudge pops, fruit bars, sherbet, and coconut-milk- or tofu-based frozen treats, also minus added sugar. Wink frozen desserts are sugar and lactose free and come in flavors such as Cinnamon Bun, Cocoa Dough, and Iced Latte, with a single gram of Net Carbs per ½ cup.

Now that you know how easy it is to put a low-carb meal on the table, it's time to learn how to make dining out just as simple and pleasurable. As you'll see in the next chapter, as long as you're prepared and know which questions to ask, you should be able to pick and choose from just about any menu, whether it's a Greek diner, fast-food chain, family dining spot, or fine restaurant. But first I want to introduce you to Joe Z., a tae kwon do champion and trainer who had nonetheless let himself become obese. More than 200 pounds lighter after adopting the Atkins Diet, Joe has rediscovered his self-esteem and found his mission in life: to inspire others to adopt a healthy lifestyle.

FROM DENIAL TO ACCOUNTABILITY

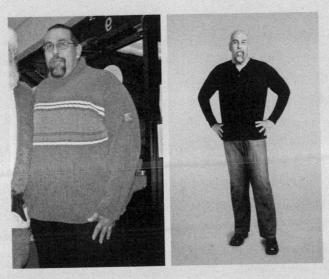

VITAL STATS

Daily Net Carb intake: 60 grams

Age: 52

Height: 6'2"

Before weight: 440 pounds

After weight: 232 pounds

Weight lost: 208 pounds

Imagine tipping the scale at 440 pounds while teaching tae kwon do in your own school! Six years ago Sacramento, California, resident Joe Z. was living a life full of such contradictions. He was also suffering constant back and knee pain and taking Motrin and Vicodin, along with cortisone injections, to try to alleviate it. And by the way, that weight is an estimate, since Joe couldn't find a scale that went that high! What is a fact is that he's now almost half the size he was. Let's hear it from Joe.

I was in complete denial. I grew up in a Latino family eating lots of beans, rice, and tortillas. I had been a jock in high school, playing on the football, tennis, and wrestling teams. I was always a big guy, and somehow I convinced myself that my 56-inch waist wasn't that different from its former 36 inches. When I was teaching a class, I'd look in the mirror and see a thin person. Then in 2007 I was watching a video of the tae kwon do world championship and I saw someone familiar on an escalator in front of one of my students. I suddenly realized that huge old guy was me!

I had been so unhappy and depressed that all I wanted to do was hide and eat. When I wasn't working, I'd barricade myself in the bedroom with snack food and watch television, which certainly didn't help my marriage. I often asked myself, "How could I have gotten so out of shape?" Of course, my eating habits were terrible. I'd either skip breakfast or hit the drive-through for fast food. Lunch was two entrées and two sets of sides, followed by an afternoon snack and an energy drink. I'd drink sugary sodas all day and then go by a fast-food place on the way home for dinner.

I could no longer do the simple kicks to demonstrate techniques to my students. At night, I snored like a freight train. After glimpsing myself on that video, I finally decided to take control of my life. Previously, I'd tried fen-phen, Weight Watchers, Medifast, and Nutrisystem, among others. I'd lose 50 pounds, feel good, and then gain back 70 pounds. I started my weight-loss journey on January 1, 2008, as part of a New Year's resolution after reading the Atkins books.

I stayed in Induction for about six months, during which my youngest daughter, who was then a senior in high school, was my Atkins buddy. During this time, my marriage fell apart, but I stayed with Atkins for two and a half years, ultimately losing 220 pounds.

Six years later I continue to avoid sugar, pasta, grains, white potatoes, and soda. I drink tea without sweetener. If I eat fast food, it's a burger without a bun. When I go to a restaurant I have a salad with chicken or meat and bring my own dressing. I love to cook, and everything I make is low in carbs. My portions are about the size of my fist. Speaking of fists, when I look at my hands today, I don't recognize them. Even my formerly wide feet are now thin. I had no idea how good it could feel to be pain free and fit into clothes I thought I could never wear. And with my blood pressure at 110/68, my doctor says I'm a new man.

But those aren't even the biggest changes. As the weight came off, my self-esteem improved. My goal has changed from losing weight to becoming as healthy as possible. I've run my first 5-kilometer race and I'm in a weight-training program. Ironically, now that I'm trying to build muscle I welcome the 12 pounds I've added! I only wish I'd started weight training earlier to improve muscle tone and help firm up my excess flesh. There are two other huge changes in my life. My second wife, who is a triathlete, was one of my former students. We met when I was plenty big, and when I got down to about 270 pounds, she asked me out! I've also embarked on a new career as a massage therapist.

In addition to my daughter, my success influenced my boss's mother to go on the Atkins program. My hope is to inspire other obese people to reach their weight-loss goals. I'm very active on Facebook. Parents of students and former students often ask for advice on how to eat and cook. I meet regularly with a group of overweight people to talk and work out together. One of the things I tell them is that at some point you have to look in the mirror and say, "I'm the one doing this to myself."

MAKE IT EASY

Don't get obsessed with a certain number. And don't panic when you hit a plateau. I sometimes lost no weight for three weeks at a time. —*J.Z.*

CHAPTER 10

DINE OUT WITH EASE

Now that you know that Atkins-style eating is no more complicated or time-consuming than putting together other meals, you'll be happy to hear that eating out is just as easy. Much of the advice on how to stay on Atkins on your own turf also applies to dining out. Ditto for meals eaten in the workplace, whether at a company event, in the employee cafeteria, or at your desk. Even when you're on a plane or in a hotel, it's perfectly possible to enjoy an Atkins-friendly meal. To stay in control of just about any food-related situation, it's just a matter of mental preparation and mastering a few techniques.

THE IMPORTANCE OF PLANNING AHEAD

Just as it's essential to have the right foods in your kitchen so you aren't blindsided when mealtime rolls around, planning ahead can be your salvation when it comes to meals in the outside world. Let's look at how that applies to eating in a restaurant, whether it's a white-table-cloth place or a coffee shop.

- *Vet the eatery.* Before you firm up plans or make a reservation, check out the menu online. If you have the Atkins app on your smartphone, use the Dining Out feature. If the low-carb choices are limited, you may prefer not to put yourself in that situation. No menu online? Check the yellow pages under "Restaurants," where menus often appear. Or do a stroll-by and scope out the menu posted in the window. If it's a takeout place, ask for a copy of the menu for future orders.

- *Know before you go.* Once you decide on a restaurant (or have been invited by someone else), review the menu online. Then and there, decide what to order. When you place your order, don't be swayed by what others are ordering or the specials that the waiter describes in irresistible terms.

- *Eat before you leave home.* This may sound like cleaning the house before the cleaning service arrives, but taking the edge off your hunger puts you, and not your low blood sugar, in the driver's seat when you sit down to eat. Half an Atkins bar, a chunk of cheese, a few slices of turkey breast, or another snack with protein and healthy fats is usually enough. However, if you're attending a dinner party where the meal may not be served until well after you usually eat, you might be wise to have a light meal, perhaps a salad topped with a protein source.

Your objective, of course, is to stay in control of the situation and not let such occasions become an excuse for falling off the Atkins wagon.

EAT OUT WITHOUT BLOWING IT

Fifty-seven percent of Americans eat at least one meal or snack away from home every day. Fortunately, you can eat out almost anywhere, as long as you pick and choose carefully. Regardless of cuisine or price point, all restaurants are in the service business, and making you happy increases the likelihood that you'll return. To become an informed diner:

- *Make your wishes clear.* Be sure the waitperson understands any modifications you want.
- *Take menu health claims with a large grain of salt.* There are no standards for the terms "low carb" or "healthy." Plus the latter usually refers to low fat, regardless of how much sugar is in a dish.
- *No sauce, please.* Order a dish prepared without sugar or starches. And steer clear of gravy, which is almost always thickened with flour or cornstarch.
- *No breading or butter either.* Inquire about ingredients and cooking technique. Make sure the entrée is roasted, grilled, pan-fried, or poached. Breaded or battered deep-fried dishes may contain harmful trans fats as well as mucho carbs.
- *Downsize supersized portions.* Share a dish or take half home in a doggie bag.
- *Pass on stews.* They're often full of potatoes or other starchy vegetables.
- *Avoid temptation.* Ask for olives or cut-up veggies in lieu of bread.
- *Double up.* Request a side salad or an additional serving of vegetables instead of the usual rice or potato served with the entrée. If your carb tolerance allows, ask for brown rice or another whole grain.
- *Dress down.* Avoid packaged salad dressings, which are usually full of sugar or corn syrup, and most house dressings. Instead, ask for oil and vinegar (or lemon juice).
- *Have a fallback.* If nothing on the menu seems "safe," ask for a large salad topped with salmon, chicken, or another protein source.

- *End on a low (carb) note.* A dish of berries with whipped cream or a cheese plate makes a great substitute for a high-carb dessert once you're out of Induction.

RESTAURANT ETIQUETTE

Eating out is about socializing as well as sustenance. Your pals are there to see you, not to get a lecture on how to eat or be made to feel guilty because they're digging into a humongous plate of pasta. Likewise, you can get information about ingredients and such from a waitperson without needing to expound on your eating habits. Follow these pointers:

- *Be friendly but firm.* There's no need to tell your companions why you are ordering a Greek salad instead of mac and cheese, but neither must you help them consume a loaf of Italian bread to be companionable. If asked, simply respond that you had a huge lunch, are cutting down on wheat, or are saving room for your entrée. If a friend who knows you're doing Atkins pressures you to share a decadent dessert, remind her that you're watching your weight.
- *Treat the waitstaff with patience.* Depending on the type of restaurant and the management style, the waitstaff may or may not be well informed about the ingredients in a dish. If you don't get a satisfactory answer, inquire pleasantly if you can talk to the manager or chef. With so many people suffering from food allergies, many restaurants will modify a dish or eliminate an ingredient upon request.

Your objective is always to make the best choices and know what you're eating, not to be cowed into eating something you're not comfortable with. At the same time, the last thing you want to do is make the occasion all about you and your eating habits.

TAKE CONTROL OF THE CONVERSATION

If your low-carb approach to eating provokes your fellow diners, try these gambits. Just be polite and smile nicely as you respond.

He or she says, "Relax, we're out on the town. One little bit of bread"—or pasta, or alcohol, or dessert—"isn't going to kill you."

- Don't respond, "Don't you realize this is a one-way ticket to the blood sugar roller coaster?"
- Instead say, "Thanks, but I'm watching my carbs right now."

He or she says, "Let's share that chocolate lava cake."

- Don't respond, "It's full of sugar, and sugar might as well be poison."
- Instead say, "I wish I could, but I fear that if I start eating it, I won't be able to stop and there'll be none for you!"

He or she says, "Let's order a couple of pizzas for everyone."

- Don't respond, "Don't you know they're made with white flour, which contains about as many nutrients as the pizza box?"
- Instead say, "You know I love pizza and I love eating with you guys, so go ahead, but I'll order a big salad."

FAST FOOD, YOUR WAY

It can be hard to avoid the major chains when you're on the road, grabbing lunch between appointments, or taking the family out without breaking the bank. Yes, fast food is convenient and inexpensive, but most offerings are full of empty carbs: in the bun, crust, breading, and condiments, and of course in the fries. Plus the beverages and condiments are full of sugar and the portions of everything are enormous.

That said, take the trouble to find the options that are more accept-able than others. Some chains boast bunless burgers and other offer-ings. Almost every major chain, and even some of the regional ones, provides extensive nutritional information on its website so you know how many carbs are in most offerings. Some even allow you to add or subtract the bun or/and condiments and immediately see the nutri-tional impact. For example, remove the bun and a Whopper goes from 51 to 3 grams of Net Carbs. In some cases you'll have to calculate Net Carbs by subtracting fiber content. Unfortunately, it's often difficult to tell whether sugar is integral or added, or whether there's sugar in one salad dressing but not another. A few general tips:

- As usual, avoid anything battered, breaded, or deep-fried. Most chicken chains now offer a grilled, broiled, or roasted alterna-tive. Pass on buttermilk biscuits, fries, and mashed potatoes as well.
- Watch out for sauces and salad dressings that contain added sugar or corn syrup. Your best bets are usually vinaigrette, ranch, and blue cheese dressings.
- Some chains let you order a burger wrapped in lettuce leaves. If not, simply remove the bun and ask for a fork.
- Most chains now offer main-dish salads with ham or chicken. However, not every salad is necessarily low in carbs. Check the nutritional profile to be sure.
- Select beverages made with noncaloric sweeteners.

Our suggestions on what to order and what to avoid at twelve na-tional chains follow. Again, the best approach is to check the menu online, make up your mind before you go, and stick to your guns.

Arby's is primarily about roasted meat and poultry sandwiches, so if you order a chicken, turkey, ham, beef, corned beef, or BLT sandwich, you'll have to remove the bun, submarine roll, or biscuit. Or order the roast chopped turkey salad with ranch dressing, which clocks in at 7 grams of Net Carbs. Website: arbys.com.

A&W menu items mostly come on burger buns or are breaded. Ditch the bun and have a hot dog, or a burger or cheeseburger with tomato and lettuce. Or order the grilled (not the crispy) chicken with ranch dipping sauce. Again, go bunless. Wash it down with A&W's sugar-free root beer. Website: awrestaurants.com.

Blimpie is also basically a sandwich shop. Again, make a meal from cheesesteak, hot pastrami, or antipasto sandwich fillings minus the bun. Or have a buffalo chicken or grilled chicken Caesar salad with blue cheese or buttermilk ranch dressing, neither of which has added sugar. Other acceptable options (although not necessarily for all Atkins phases) include tuna salad, chicken gumbo, cream of broccoli soup, beef stew, and Yankee pot roast. Website: blimpie.com.

Burger King. Again, lose the bun, and most burgers, Whoppers, and the broiled chicken patty pass muster. Salads are usually full of high-carb additions, but two exceptions are the Chicken BLT and Caesar Garden Fresh Salads. Be sure to order either with the grilled (not fried) chicken, remove the croutons, and top with Ken's ranch dressing. Website: bk.com.

Carl's Jr. actually offers low-carb choices, including the Low-Carb Six-Dollar Burger (wrapped in lettuce leaves) and the (bunless) Low-Carb Charbroiled Chicken Club. Other options minus the bun that pass muster: the Famous Star, Big Carl, Guacamole Bacon Burger, and most other burgers and cheeseburgers. Or order the Charbroiled Chicken Salad but lose the croutons. House and blue cheese salad dressings are sugar free, as are the house and buffalo wing sauces. Website: carlsjr.com.

Chick-fil-A has some acceptable options once you remove the biscuit or bread on the breakfast egg, cheese, sausage, and bacon dishes. Or unwrap and discard the tortilla on the sausage break-fast burrito. Skip the breaded chicken and order a Chargrilled Chicken Club or Chicken Salad sandwich (minus the bread) or a Chargrilled Chicken Garden or Southwest Chargrilled Salad. Top with blue cheese, Caesar, or buttermilk ranch salad dressing. Website: chick-fil-a.com.

Dairy Queen. It's possible to fuel up here with a burger, cheeseburger, hot dog, cheese dog, or grilled chicken or turkey sandwich, minus the bun. BBQ, Wild Buffalo, and ranch dipping sauces are acceptable, as is the side salad. Website: dairyqueen.com.

Hardee's also has some low-carb specialties. Try the Low-Carb Thickburger or the Charbroiled Chicken Club "Sandwich," wrapped in lettuce leaves. Website: hardees.com.

KFC offers at least one acceptable dish, the Kentucky Grilled Chicken. Pass on the biscuits and mashed potatoes; instead, have a side of green beans. Website: kfc.com.

McDonald's burgers and cheeseburgers are fine "naked," as is the grilled chicken club, the Premium Bacon Ranch or Caesar salad with or without grilled chicken, and scrambled eggs and sausage patties. Ask for Newman's Own Creamy Caesar Dressing. Website: mcdonalds.com.

Subway subs can be ordered as a salad (request no croutons), including the cold cut combo, Subway Club, tuna fish, BLT, Black Forest ham, turkey breast, and roast beef. Also okay are the vinaigrette dressing and omelets minus the sandwich. Website: subwayfreshbuzz.com.

Wendy's. Once more, say bye-bye to the bun and have the rest of any burger or cheeseburger; also okay are the chicken BLT or the Caesar salad (omit croutons) with Ultimate Chicken Grill Fillet and Supreme Caesar Dressing. Website: wendys.com.

CASUAL DINING, YOUR WAY

When you're not in the mood for fast food but don't want to make a big dent in your wallet, there's another kind of chain restaurant you can patronize. Casual dining restaurants such as Chipotle, TGI Friday, and Ruby Tuesday also offer more choices and opportunities to "have it your way" in terms of sauces, fixings, cheeses, and add-ons for burgers, chicken, steaks, salads, and other entrées. However, you'll still have to be alert for the same minefield of monster portions, sauces and dressings full of sugar, and a bevy of battered and breaded dishes. Most of these eateries have lengthy menus, and among the sea of high-carb options you can find some Atkins-friendly items. You may want to ask that half the meal be put in a doggie bag *before* you begin, so you can have it for lunch the next day. Let's visit a few of the more popular casual dining chains.

Applebee's has some Atkins-friendly appetizers, including classic wings with classic buffalo sauce. Then move on to New York strip steak or the steak and grilled shrimp combo. You can order any entrée without sides and then add the ones you prefer. How about a topper of grilled onions or sautéed garlic mushrooms and a seasonal berry and spinach salad? Website: applebees.com.

Baja Fresh offers the option of "bare burritos" served over a bed of chopped romaine instead of in a tortilla. Skip the Baja Bowls, which include white rice, but if you remove the tortillas from any other salad you should be good to go. Or put together a meal from several sides, such as guacamole; salsa; mixed grilled peppers, chiles, and onion; and grilled wahoo (a type of fish). Website: bajafresh.com.

Chili's has decided that bigger is not always better, and now suggests that a pair of diners share an appetizer and then a couple of entrées. How about grilled chicken salad, grilled salmon with garlic and herbs, margarita-grilled chicken, Monterey chicken, or Spicy Garlic and Lime-Grilled Shrimp? Website: chilis.com.

Chipotle Mexican Grill has a menu heavy on tortillas, but you can put together your own salad on a base of romaine tossed with vinaigrette. Choose from grilled chicken, steak, fish, or beef, and top it with veggies, salsa, cheese, sour cream, or guacamole for a great salad containing about 10 grams of Net Carbs. Website: chipotle.com.

Olive Garden takes Italian cuisine beyond pasta and breaded entrées. Try Mussels di Napoli, Shrimp Scampi, Herb-Grilled Salmon, Mixed Grill, or one of several steak dishes—skip the potatoes, if necessary, for these last two. Or fall back on the Grilled Chicken Caesar Salad—just remove the croutons. Website: olivegarden.com.

Outback Steakhouse isn't just about steak. Grilled Norwegian salmon or shrimp (hot off the barbie), seared ahi tuna, and the Outback special 6-ounce steak will barely make a dent in your daily carb budget. Grilled asparagus makes a great side dish. In the mood for a hearty salad? Try the Classic Wedge Blue Cheese Salad. Website: outback.com.

Ruby Tuesday helps put you in the driver's seat. Assemble a main-dish salad from a long list of fresh ingredients, or pick from a host of veggie sides to go with your entrée. Although the menu is studded with breaded and fried dishes, there are also many you can pick from, such as "fresh-crafted" burgers, grilled salmon, chicken fresco, petite sirloin and lobster tail, and jumbo skewered shrimp. Website: rubytuesday.com.

TGI Friday's offers huge portions, lots of choices, and many Atkins–friendly dishes. Try the Bacon and Bleu Sirloin or Grilled Salmon with Langostino Lobster, with either Ginger Lime Slaw or the Tomato Mozzarella Salad. The grilled chicken Cobb salad is also a safe bet. Website: tgifridays.com.

NAVIGATING DIFFICULT SITUATIONS

Some places pose more of a challenge to Atkins followers than others. And sometimes the best alternative is still not ideal, but hey, we live in the real world. So let's scope out what your best choices are at pizza parlors, coffee shops, vending machines, convenience stores, and more.

- *A pizza parlor.* Yes, you can resort to the old (and messy) trick of scraping the toppings off the pizza crust, but instead, order an antipasto plate or a salad topped with grilled chicken. If pizza is the only thing on the menu, opt for a thin-crust version, preferably made with whole wheat.

- *A coffee shop.* Whether it's Starbucks or a local joint (or even a coffee cart), order hot or iced coffee, black or with cream or half-and-half, rather than any of the sugar-laden concoctions. Instead of cappuccino, order caffè breve, made with espresso and half-and-half (instead of milk), a mocha breve, or an iced breve.

- *Vending machines.* Even offerings promoted as "healthful" are made with sugar and white flour. Opt for a bag of peanuts, pumpkin seeds, or other nuts or seeds, or have some sugar-free jerky. Although more machines now offer light meals to heat up in the microwave, they're usually based on noodles or rice, so give them a pass.

- *Gas station convenience stores.* The pickings can be pretty slim here, but possibilities include string cheese, sugar-free jerky, peanut butter, fresh fruit, a small container of plain whole-milk yogurt, nuts or seeds, and popcorn.

MOBILE FOOD

No time to sit down when your lunch hour is spent running errands or hitting the gym? Food carts to the rescue, and nowadays they're selling not just hot dogs and pizza, but also a host of other ethnic specialties. As food suitable for a quick bite or a meal on the run, however, most rely upon a tortilla, roll, waffle, empanada, or pizza crust to contain the other ingredients. Nonetheless, you may be able to deconstruct street food to make it Atkins friendly. Ask if you can have it on a plate instead, but don't be surprised if the vendor can't do that. If you're heading back to your workplace, when you get there simply remove the bun, pita, rice, or other high-carb ingredient. Among the United Nations of possibilities, here are just a few:

- *American classics.* BBQ carts offer a variety of smoked ribs, beef brisket, chicken parts, pork loin, link sausages, and blackened catfish with sides. The Philadelphia cheesesteak sandwich contains tender beef strips grilled with peppers and onions, topped with melted American cheese, and served on a hoagie roll, which you can ditch.
- *Argentinean.* This cuisine is big on beef, but you're likely to find it stuffed into an empanada with onions, peppers, and potatoes.
- *Cambodian.* Lemongrass skewered chicken, pork stew with hard-boiled eggs, and grilled short ribs are all typical dishes, usually served on rice.
- *Caribbean.* Usually served in a flatbread called a roti or over rice, curries are big in this cuisine; they are often served with a salad.
- *Greek or Middle Eastern.* Have kebabs, a lamb or chicken gyro, or falafel with lettuce, tomato, hummus, and cucumbers.
- *Korean.* Rice or noodles turn up in almost every dish. Simply eat the rest and leave them. Better yet, try a bento box of grilled marinated chicken and steamed veggies. The street dish of

Korea, bi bim bop, is rice topped with sautéed seasoned veggies, your choice of meat, and a fried egg.

You can eat Atkins style in almost any restaurant if you know what to order. Some cuisines, such as Greek or Korean, are highly compatible with a low-carb lifestyle. Mexican and Chinese are a bit more difficult to navigate. However, in almost every case, there are Atkins-appropriate choices.

DINING OUT, ITALIAN STYLE

Italian food is a lot more than the pizza and pasta with red sauce that hail from southern Italy. Northern Italian food features rich butter and cream sauces, and the signature element in Florentine dishes is spinach. There are three basic secrets to enjoying the food at an Italian restaurant while complying with Atkins:

- Avoid the usual sides of spaghetti, polenta, or risotto.
- Ask for a bowl of olives as a starter in lieu of garlic bread.
- Ask whether dishes such as veal marsala or veal Florentine are breaded. Some chefs bread them; others don't.

Here are other ways to keep the carbs down:

HAVE THIS	INSTEAD OF THAT
Seafood salad	Battered and fried calamari
Mixed grilled vegetables or portobello mushrooms	Fried mozzarella sticks
Salad of arugula, fennel, and shaved Parmesan	Garlic bread
Antipasto platter	Stuffed clams
Escarole or stracciatella soup	Fettuccini Alfredo
Roasted or grilled seafood	Linguini with clam sauce
Grilled chicken breast or pork loin	Any risotto dish
Veal piccata or scaloppini	Veal or eggplant Parmesan

DINING OUT, GREEK STYLE

Greek food is based on olives, olive oil, lemons, eggplant, zucchini, spinach, fennel, grape leaves, yogurt, garlic, mint, dill, rosemary, and tahini (ground sesame seeds). Whether at a Greek diner or an elegant restaurant, fresh fish is always a good choice. The predominant meat is lamb, but beef also appears on the menu. Request another vegetable instead of rice or flatbread. Greek salads are full of good things, including feta cheese, olives, tomatoes, and fresh basil. Steer clear of filo (phyllo), paper-thin sheets of pastry dough used in the dessert called baklava as well as in savory dishes such as spanakopita. To keep the carbs down:

HAVE THIS	INSTEAD OF THAT
Tzatziki (yogurt, cucumber, and garlic dip)	Skordalia (thick potato-garlic spread)
Avgolemono (chicken soup with egg and lemon)	Spanakopita or tyropita
Fresh vegetables and taramosalata (creamy fish roe spread)	Dolmades (stuffed grape leaves)
Beef or lamb souvlaki	Moussaka
Braised lamb shanks	Pastitsio with pasta
Chicken grilled with lemon, garlic, and herbs	Chicken pilaf
Grilled prawns, octopus, or swordfish	Fried calamari
Cheese plate	Baklava

DINING OUT, MIDDLE EASTERN STYLE

Garlic, onions, cardamom, coriander, sesame, cumin, thyme, marjoram, and sumac are the predominant seasonings used with lamb and other meats. Many dishes, such as shish kebab and baklava, are also found in Greek cuisine. Baba ganoush, similar to hummus, is made of roasted eggplant mashed and mixed with garlic and tahini. Traditionally, baba ganoush is eaten with flatbread, but celery sticks or green pepper chunks make fine substitutes. More ways to keep the carbs down:

HAVE THIS	INSTEAD OF THAT
Loubieh (green beans with tomatoes)	Tabbouleh (bulgur salad)
Eggplant with garlic, tomatoes, and peppers	Fattoush (bread, cucumber, and tomato salad)
Lamb shish kebab	Kibbe (ground lamb and bulgur patty)
Kofta (skewered and grilled ground lamb and onion patties)	Falafel (deep-fried chickpea patties)
Shish taouk (skewered and marinated chicken pieces grilled over charcoal)	B'steeya (Moroccan chicken pie with almonds)

DINING OUT, MEXICAN STYLE

Genuine Mexican cuisine is far more subtle and varied than the Tex-Mex, New Mexican style, and Cal-Mex variations that usually pass for Mexican cuisine in the United States. Garlic, chiles, cilantro, and cumin are common denominators. Fortunately, tortillas, beans, and rice are just the tip of the culinary iceberg. For starters, you can't go wrong with guacamole and salsa made without added sugar. If you're a fan of enchiladas verdes, tortillas filled with spiced chicken and covered with a tangy green sauce of tomatillos and cilantro, just ask for the chicken filling minus the tortillas and topped with the sauce. Beef, chicken, or shrimp fajitas are seared in a skillet with sliced onions and peppers. Just pass on the tortillas, yellow rice, and refried beans. For other ways to keep the carbs down:

HAVE THIS	INSTEAD OF THAT
Jicama sticks	Tortilla chips
Grilled chicken wings	Stuffed jalapeño peppers or chiles rellenos
Jicama salad	Nachos
Sopa de albondigas (meatball and vegetable soup)	Quesadillas
Grilled fish (pescado)	Taco, tamale, or enchilada platter
Pollo asado (grilled chicken)	Chimichangas or flautas

| Chicken or turkey mole (a complex sauce made with ground cocoa beans) | Chicken tortillas |
| Camarones al ajillo (shrimp in garlic sauce) | Shrimp enchiladas |

DINING OUT, FRENCH STYLE

Choose carefully and make a few modifications, and there are plenty of Atkins-friendly dishes in French cuisine. You'll find fish, herbs, and olives in dishes that hail from Provence; butter and apples in those from Normandy; stews simmered in wine from Burgundy and Bordeaux; and sausages and beer in Alsatian specialties. Hollandaise and many other classic French sauces are based on butter or olive oil and thickened with egg yolks rather than flour. Other tips to curb the carbs: order French onion soup with Gruyère cheese, but without the toasted bread, and push the potatoes in coq au vin to the side of your plate.

HAVE THIS	INSTEAD OF THAT
Frisée salad with bacon and a poached egg	Alsatian tart (bacon, onion, and egg pie)
Coquilles St. Jacques (scallops in cream sauce topped with cheese)	Lobster in puff pastry
Mussels in white wine sauce or bouillabaisse (fish stew)	Vichyssoise (cream of leek and potato soup)
Coq au vin	Duck à l'orange or aux cerises
Entrecôte or tournedos Bordelaise (steak in shallot and red wine sauce)	Croque monsieur (fried ham and cheese sandwich)
Veal Marengo	Veal Prince Orloff
Cheese plate	Crêpes Suzette

DINING OUT, INDIAN STYLE

Indian food comprises a varied collection of regional cuisines. Although many dishes rely on rice and other grains, you'll also find lamb, duck, pork, and even goat on the menu. The typical Indian menu offers many choices that provide a good balance of protein and fiber-rich vegetables. Just stay away from breads, rice, and other starchy dishes. Tandoori dishes are the most popular Indian offerings in this country, followed by curries. You'll also find grilled kebabs and dals, which are lentil, chickpea, or bean dishes. Try raita, which is yogurt mixed with minced cucumbers, to ease the heat of some of the hotter curries. To cut the carbs:

HAVE THIS	INSTEAD OF THAT
Shahi paneer (cheese in a creamy curried tomato sauce)	Vegetable samosas (savory pastries)
Roasted eggplant with onions and spices	Pakora (fritters)
Chicken shorba	Mulligatawny soup
Tandoori chicken or other meat	Vindaloo (contains potatoes)
Korma (meat in a cream sauce)	Biryani (a rice dish)
Chicken, fish, or meat curry	Dal
Chicken, lamb, or shrimp kebabs	Chicken or lamb saag

DINING OUT, CHINESE STYLE

Rice and noodles are the staples of the four major regional cuisines: Cantonese, Szechuan, Hunan, and Shandong. Most dishes use meat or fish as an addition rather than the main ingredient and rely on a sauce—generally thickened with cornstarch. If possible, request that any dish be prepared with the sauce on the side. Wu shu duck, for example, is usually dusted with almond flour, fried, and served with a dark brown sauce. The sauce is sweetened, but the duck itself is delicious without it. Avoid any sweet-and-sour and breaded or battered dishes as well as noodle dishes. A small portion of brown rice is fine, if your carb tolerance allows. Have Peking duck and mu shu pork but skip the pancakes and plum sauce. To avoid empty carbs:

HAVE THIS	INSTEAD OF THAT
Clear egg drop soup (without cornstarch)	Fried wontons
Hot-and-sour soup	Egg roll
Sizzling shrimp platter	Shrimp fried rice
Steamed or stir-fried tofu with vegetables	Deep-fried tofu dishes
Beef with Chinese mushrooms	Any noodle-based dish
Stir-fried pork with garlic sauce	Sweet-and-sour pork
Peking duck	General Tso's chicken

DINING OUT, JAPANESE STYLE

White rice is a staple of this cuisine, but you can still enjoy Japanese food without it. Sauces and seasonings include shoyu, or Japanese soy sauce; mirin, sweet rice wine that usually contains added sugar; dashi, broth made from dried fish (bonito) flakes; ponzu, a dipping sauce made from shoyu, rice wine vinegar, dashi, and seaweed; wasabi, an extremely hot Japanese horseradish; pickled ginger; miso, a paste made from fermented soybeans; and sesame seeds and toasted sesame oil. A variety of vegetables are usually grilled or blanched briefly. Try burdock (a relative of the artichoke), daikon, lotus root, and Japanese eggplant. Also sample the pickled vegetables, including seaweed, which are most often served as a snack or appetizer. *Oshinko* means "pickle" in Japanese, but these are unlike any gherkins you've ever tried. For a fun-to-eat, satisfying main course, try shabu-shabu, thin slices of beef and vegetables that you cook at the table in broth—it's the Japanese version of fondue. To cut the carbs:

HAVE THIS	INSTEAD OF THAT
Sashimi	Sushi
Oshinko, edamame, steamed vegetables, or grilled eggplant	Gyoza (fried vegetable dumplings)
Shabu-shabu	Sukiyaki
Broiled fish or shrimp with soy or ginger sauce	Shrimp tempura

Grilled squid	Seafood noodle dishes
Negamaki (scallions wrapped in thin-sliced beef) dipped in soy sauce	Beef teriyaki (contains added sugar)

DINING OUT, THAI STYLE

Pad thai, the national dish, is based on noodles with shrimp, scallions, eggs, dried tofu, bean sprouts, and chopped peanuts. But the flavors and combinations that make Thai food distinctive, including coconut milk, lemongrass, tamarind, cilantro, turmeric, cumin, chiles, lime juice, and kaffir lime leaves, can be found in many other dishes. For example, nua yang nam tok is made with sliced steak marinated in lime juice and mixed with chiles, onion, tomato, cucumber, coriander leaves, and lettuce. The same flavors are applied to sliced squid in yum pla muk. Try tom yum goong, a shrimp soup with straw mushrooms, seasoned with lime juice, lemongrass, and hot peppers; or gai tom kha, made with chicken slices in coconut milk. In general, it's best to stick to dishes that are quickly sautéed with vegetables and aromatic Thai herbs. To keep a lid on carbs:

HAVE THIS	INSTEAD OF THAT
Tom yum goong	Dumplings or spring rolls
Sautéed shrimp with basil, chiles, and onion	Pad thai
Sautéed scallops with mushrooms, zucchini, and chili paste	Curried scallops with potatoes
Sautéed shrimp with shrimp paste and green beans	Sautéed shrimp with black bean sauce
Sautéed mixed vegetables	Fried rice

DINING OUT, KOREAN STYLE

Fish and shellfish, usually grilled or stewed in a sauce, make up a large part of the typical Korean diet. Pork, beef, and chicken are often marinated and grilled. Some dishes, such as kalbi tang, a marinated beef rib stew, are served with rice; others come with noodles. Korea is also known for its barbecue (bulgogi) of thin slices of a premium cut of beef. A Korean restaurant may also offer barbecued chicken and pork, and perhaps fish and squid bulgogi, but skip the sauce, which is likely sweetened with sugar. Kimchi, an assortment of fermented vegetables seasoned with hot chiles, salt, garlic, onions, ginger, and oyster or fish sauce, is one of the best-known Korean specialties. To keep carbs under control:

HAVE THIS	INSTEAD OF THAT
Cold tofu	Pa jon (scallion pancake)
Twoenjangguk (soup of fermented soybean paste and baby clams)	Korean dumplings
Shinsollo (hot pot of meat or fish, vegetables, and tofu)	Any rice dish
Any barbecued dish	Any rice or noodle dish

BE ON YOUR *GUEST* BEHAVIOR

Dining at a friend or relative's house should be an enjoyable occasion. But you may fear that your host or hostess will be offended if you don't eat everything, exclaim how fabulous it is, and ask for seconds. What to do if you know that some of the dishes aren't going to pass muster carbwise? To a large degree, it depends on the circumstances.

- *The meal is buffet style.* You're in luck. Simply pick the items you can eat and pass on the others. If people are sitting all over the house or yard, it's unlikely your host will notice what each guest selects.
- *The invitation says potluck.* Bring a low-carb dish and share it. Also have suitable foods prepared by others, such as salad or vegetables.

- *It's a sit-down affair.* Your host and/or hostess are in charge, and your relationship with them is more important than avoiding a few grams of added sugar or a spoonful of potatoes au gratin. That doesn't mean that you're not within your rights to ask for sauce on the side or for a small portion of a high-carb dish. When it comes to dessert, ask for a small piece, take a bite, and leave the rest on the plate.

Many people have food allergies or dietary preferences. If your host had to accommodate the personal food issues of every guest, he or she might never get a meal on the table! However, if you're asked before the event whether there's anything you don't eat, you certainly can say that you're slimming down and are staying away from desserts and starches. Immediately add that by no means should that influence the menu. Instead, just eat the main dish and vegetables.

EATING ON THE ROAD

When you're on your own turf, it's always easier to stick to your usual routine. If you travel for business or pleasure, your usual patterns may be disrupted by time zone changes, a schedule you don't control, or countless other factors. Before you leave the house:

- If you have to be up at dawn, grab an Atkins bar or prepare a low-carb breakfast for yourself the night before. Have it before you go or take it with you. Don't leave home empty-handed or on an empty stomach.
- Know where to find acceptable snacks or meals so that if you can't bring something with you, at least you know the location of a convenience store or fast-food place with low-carb options along the way.

- One item will do as a snack, but if you're putting together a meal, you'll need to include several items. Pack each item in a separate resealable bag in an insulated carrier.
- Bring suitable foods such as the ones listed as snacks appropriate for the various phases (see pages 87, 137, and 168) to keep you satisfied and able to resist temptation.

If you're on vacation and sightseeing or engaging in activities such as hiking, swimming, or skiing, chances are you're getting plenty of exercise. But if you're spending most of your waking hours in a conference room or driving from one appointment to another, you'll probably want to find a way to get in some physical activity. Many hotels have a fitness center; if not, you can always bring your walking shoes and get out and explore the surroundings.

ON THE WING

Your commitment to eating the Atkins way needn't be disrupted en route if you follow these suggestions for a smooth flight.

- Atkins bars are great portable snacks—just don't try to carry a shake on a plane! (Like all beverages, it can't go through security.)
- Bring suitable food from home packed in a way that will pass muster at security.
- Alternatively, after security clearance, visit a salad bar. Pile up the greens and top them with slices of chicken or another protein source to take with you on the plane. Also purchase bottled water, club soda, unsweetened tea, coffee, or herb tea so that you can stay hydrated in the air.
- Go to the website for the carrier you're flying on and check out the meal options to ensure that something suitable is available. Most airlines have a main-dish salad that will serve.
- Bring small bags of nuts or seeds with you to munch on.

LOW-CARB ROOM SERVICE

Staying in a hotel can be a nice break from your usual responsibilities. No need to make dinner—or the bed! But the room's refrigerator is likely full of the same high-carb foods you've banished from your own kitchen: cookies, candy, crackers, and chips. If you fear that you'll be tempted, decline the key to the fridge or return it to the front desk. (And there's no need to spend $5 for a bottle of water, even if you are on an expense account!) Room service is wonderfully convenient, but it too poses some challenges:

- Specify what you *don't* want—no toast, bread, or jam, for example as well as what you *do* want.
- Have the server immediately remove anything you don't want tempting you if it arrives despite your instructions.
- As soon as you've eaten, put the tray outside the door.

Whether you're eating out, traveling, or grabbing a meal during your lunch break, with this wealth of information you'll undoubtedly feel more in control of your meals away from home. In the next chapter, I hope to lure you back into your own kitchen to try out some delicious quick and easy Atkins recipes, all of which are acceptable from day one on Atkins.

RECIPES

RECIPE INDEX

BREAKFASTS

LUNCH OR DINNER DISHES

SAUCES

MAIN DISH SALADS

SOUPS, CHOWDERS, AND CHILI

SNACKS

DESSERTS

COOK'S NOTES

Most of the ingredients found in the following recipes are available in your supermarket or a shopping club. Sources for a few less familiar ingredients are provided.

Several of the recipes call for coconut-flax flour blend. To make, mix equal parts coconut flour with ground flaxseed and refrigerate in an airtight container. Both ingredients can be found in most supermarkets in the baking aisle or gluten-free section, as well as at Walmart and natural foods stores. (Bob's Red Mill is one good brand.) If you opt to use only ground flaxseed in baked goods, the texture will not be as cakelike and some people find the taste bitter. For best results, flaxseed should be finely ground in a coffee grinder or mini food processor; most preground brands are chunky. The coconut-flax flour blend also dials down the carbs but preserves a soft cakelike texture.

Some recipes call for tamari, which contains no wheat, rather than soy sauce, which does. However, if you have no tamari on hand, feel free to substitute soy sauce.

Some recipes call for both cooking spray (use the canola or olive oil kind) *and* oil or butter. Use the cooking spray first to lubricate the pan, which enables the oil or butter to spread more evenly, reducing the risk of items such as crêpes sticking to the pan.

Nutritionals per serving have been rounded off to the nearest whole gram, which is why occasionally the total carbs minus fiber may not appear to compute. Also provided is the number of grams of foundation vegetables in each serving. We used stevia to calculate nutritionals; other acceptable sweeteners include sucralose, saccharin, xylitol, and maltitol, as well as a new entry, lo han gua, made from an extract of monk fruit.

All recipes are acceptable for Phases 1 to 4. If a variation is suitable only for later phases, that is indicated. Note that the inclusion of nuts and seeds in Phase 1 is acceptable in both Atkins products and recipes if the Net Carb count is appropriate for this phase, because nuts and seeds do not provoke a blood sugar response.

Recipes are coded as follows:

7   No more than seven ingredients (plus salt and pepper)

🕐   Total prep time of 20 minutes or less

▤   Do-ahead recipes that can be refrigerated or frozen

    Can be made in a slow cooker

BREAKFASTS

Zucchini-Pumpkin Spice Pancakes ◐ ▤

Zucchini and pumpkin make great desserts and breakfast fare. Top with sugar-free breakfast syrup and/or a dollop of mascarpone cheese. Allow leftover pancakes to cool completely, wrap individually in plastic wrap, and freeze for up to 3 months. Reheat in a toaster oven for 10 minutes or in a preheated 300°F oven for 15 minutes. Be sure to use plain canned pumpkin, not pumpkin pie filling, which is full of sugar.

Makes: 4 (3-pancake) servings
Active Time: 10 minutes
Total Time: 40 minutes

4 large eggs, separated

½ small zucchini, grated (about 1 cup)

½ cup canned pumpkin

½ cup plain unsweetened soy milk

1 teaspoon acceptable sweetener

¼ cup coconut-flax flour blend

2 tablespoons plain unsweetened protein powder

¼ teaspoon salt

½ teaspoon baking powder

½ teaspoon pumpkin pie spice mix

Canola or olive oil cooking spray

4 teaspoons canola oil

1. In a large mixing bowl and using an electric mixer at high speed, beat the egg whites until stiff peaks form, about 1 minute. Set aside.
2. Place the egg yolks, zucchini, pumpkin, soy milk, and sweetener in another large bowl and stir well.
3. Combine the coconut-flax flour blend, protein powder, salt, baking powder, and pumpkin pie spice in a medium bowl and stir well. (Or mix on a sheet of wax paper to avoid having to wash another bowl.)

4. Sprinkle dry mixture over the egg yolk mixture and add ¼ cup of the beaten egg whites. Fold until combined. Fold in the remaining egg whites until the mixture is light and fluffy.

5. Coat a large skillet or pancake griddle with cooking spray and place it over medium heat. Add 1 teaspoon oil. Using a ¼-cup measure, drop 3 mounds of batter into the skillet, and smooth out with the back of a spoon. Cook 2–3 minutes, until edges are slightly browned. Flip and cook 2–3 minutes more, until firm in the middle. Transfer to a plate and repeat three times with remaining pancake batter, using 1 teaspoon canola oil each time. Serve immediately.

PER SERVING: Net Carbs: 4 grams; Total Carbs: 8 grams; Fiber: 4 grams; Protein: 14 grams;
Fat: 13 grams; Calories: 198; Foundation Vegetables Net Carbs: 2 grams

VARIATIONS

- In place of the coconut-flax flour blend, use ¼ cup finely ground flaxseed.
- Swap yellow summer squash for zucchini.
- Phases 3 and 4: Substitute grated apple—no need to peel it—for zucchini.

Eggs Parmesan

To make this one-dish meal an equally tasty lunch or light dinner, add sausages or bacon. Serve with your favorite hot sauce, if you wish.

Makes: 4 servings
Active Time: 10 minutes
Total Time: 15 minutes

1 tablespoon virgin olive oil

3 cups broccoli florets, roughly chopped

½ cup jarred or canned tomato sauce

4 large eggs

½ cup grated mozzarella

1 cup finely grated Parmesan cheese

Salt and freshly ground pepper

1. Heat a large skillet over high heat and add the oil. Add the broccoli florets and cook 2–3 minutes, stirring frequently, until they begin to soften.
2. Turn the heat to low and spoon the tomato sauce over the broccoli. Crack the eggs over the sauce, spacing them 4 inches apart. Sprinkle with mozzarella and then Parmesan.
3. Cover and cook 4 to 5 minutes, until the cheese is melted and the whites of the eggs are cooked through but the yolks are still slightly runny.
4. Using a spatula, spoon out four portions, each with an egg in the middle, into soup bowls. Sprinkle with salt and pepper and serve immediately.

PER SERVING: Net Carbs: 4 grams; Total Carbs: 6 grams; Fiber: 2 grams; Protein: 19 grams; Fat: 17 grams; Calories: 252; Foundation Vegetables Net Carbs: 2 grams

VARIATIONS

- Substitute cauliflower for broccoli.
- In Phase 2 and beyond, slide each portion into low-carb pita.

Chocolate Waffles

The whole family will enjoy these sweet, tender waffles. Top each waffle with a dollop of whipped cream if you wish. Be sure to use unsweetened cocoa, not hot chocolate mix.

Makes: 4 (1-waffle) servings
Active Time: 10 minutes
Total Time: 30 minutes

4 large eggs, separated

¼ teaspoon salt

¾ cup plain unsweetened soy milk

½ cup mascarpone

2 tablespoons melted butter, cooled

1 teaspoon acceptable sweetener

1 teaspoon vanilla extract

¼ cup coconut-flax flour blend

2 tablespoons unsweetened protein powder

2 tablespoons unsweetened cocoa powder

½ teaspoon baking powder

Canola or olive oil cooking spray

1. In a large mixing bowl and using an electric mixer, beat the egg whites and salt on high speed until stiff peaks form. Set aside.

2. In a second large bowl, whisk egg yolks, soy milk, mascarpone, butter, sweetener, and vanilla. Add the coconut-flax flour blend, protein powder, cocoa powder, and baking powder and stir to combine.

3. Add ¼ cup beaten egg whites to the egg yolk mixture. Using a rubber spatula, fold in the egg whites and all of the flour until just combined, about 8 turns, forming a sticky mass. Fold in another ¼ cup egg whites until the mixture becomes lighter, an additional 4–5 turns. Finally, fold in the remaining egg mixture. There will be small lumps. Don't overmix.

4. Heat a waffle iron according to the manufacturer's instructions and mist with cooking spray. Add ½ cup batter and spread it evenly with the back of a spoon. Cover and cook 2–3 minutes or until the waffle is firm and light brown. Repeat with remaining batter and serve immediately. Or cool to room temperature, double-wrap in plastic wrap, and freeze.

PER SERVING: Net Carbs: 3 grams; Total Carbs: 7 grams; Fiber: 4 grams; Protein: 16 grams;

Fat: 26 grams; Calories: 326; Foundation Vegetables Net Carbs: 0 grams

VARIATIONS

- In place of the coconut-flax flour blend, use ¼ cup finely ground flaxseed.
- In Phase 2, top with fresh or frozen raspberries or strawberries.

Breakfast Casserole

Ideal for the beginner cook, this dish can be made ahead and reheated. If you're not used to cooking with greens such as kale, this rich, cheesy recipe is a great way to start. You can also serve at lunch or dinner.

Makes: 4 servings
Active Time: 10 minutes
Total Time: 35 minutes

1 tablespoon virgin olive oil

2 Italian sausage links, chopped

½ cup chopped red onion

1 8-ounce package button or cremini mushrooms, chopped

1 cup thinly sliced packed kale (stems and ribs removed)

8 large eggs, lightly beaten

1 cup grated Cheddar cheese

1 teaspoon baking powder

Salt and freshly ground black pepper

1. Preheat oven to 400°F. Warm a large skillet over medium heat. Add the olive oil, sausage, and onion. Cook 3–4 minutes, breaking up the sausage with the back of a wooden spoon as it browns. Add the mushrooms and cook 1 minute more, until they soften. Add the kale and set aside to cool for 5 minutes.
2. Meanwhile, in a large bowl, whisk eggs, cheese, and baking powder. Add the sausage mixture and transfer to an 8-inch-square baking dish lined with aluminum foil.
3. Bake uncovered 20–25 minutes, until the eggs puff up and the casserole is firm in the center. Cool 5 minutes, then slice into 4 even wedges. Season with salt and pepper and serve immediately.

PER SERVING: Net Carbs: 7 grams; Total Carbs: 6 grams; Fiber: 1 gram; Protein: 26 grams; Fat: 32 grams; Calories: 414; Foundation Vegetables Net Carbs: 5 grams

VARIATIONS

- Use crumbled bacon, cubed ham, cooked turkey cubes, or other leftovers in place of sausage.
- Substitute spinach or arugula for kale.

Breakfast Sandwich **7** ◖ ⊟

There's a surprise ingredient in this savory homemade "flatbread" that makes this sandwich a protein all-star: ground chicken! If you don't have any leftover chicken, use grilled or roasted skinless chicken cubes from the deli department. You'll find them under the Bell & Evans and Perdue labels, among others. Grind the chicken in the food processor.

Makes: 2 servings
Active Time: 10 minutes
Total Time: 25 minutes

1 large egg

½ cup ground cooked chicken

½ cup finely grated Parmesan cheese

2 tablespoons ground flaxseed

½ teaspoon Italian seasoning (optional)

Olive oil or canola oil cooking spray

2 slices cooked bacon, cut into quarters

2 slices Cheddar cheese

Salt and freshly ground black pepper

1. Preheat the oven to 450°F. Make the flatbread: In a large bowl whisk the egg. Add the ground chicken, Parmesan, flaxseed, and Italian seasoning, if using, and mix until it forms a heavy dough.
2. Coat an 8-inch-square baking dish with cooking spray. Add the dough and press it into the pan using the back of a fork, forming an even layer. The surface of the dough will have ridges.
3. Bake 8–10 minutes, until firm. Cut the flatbread into 4 even squares.

4. Layer two squares of the flatbread with bacon and top each with a slice of Cheddar cheese and then another flatbread square. Press down firmly and bake an additional 3–4 minutes, until the cheese melts.

5. Season with salt and pepper and serve immediately. Or wrap in aluminum foil to go. Reheat in a 400°F oven for 10 minutes.

PER SERVING: Net Carbs: 1 gram; Total Carbs: 2 grams; Fiber: 1 gram; Protein: 23 grams;

Fat: 17 grams; Calories: 245; Foundation Vegetables Net Carbs: 0 grams

VARIATIONS

- Instead of bacon, use a cooked sausage link, cut into 8 thin slices.
- Add leftover veggies such as sautéed spinach and/or mushrooms.
- Make crackers with the flatbread dough by following steps 1–3. Remove from the pan and cool completely on a plate before wrapping in aluminum foil and storing refrigerated for up to 4 days, or freeze for up to 3 months in a resealable bag.

LUNCH OR DINNER DISHES

Deep-Dish Sausage and Cauliflower Pizza

If you devour this delicious pizza the minute it comes out of the oven, you'll need a knife and fork. Let it cool for 10 minutes, though, and the crust will firm up, so you can use your fingers. It also keeps nicely in the fridge for up to 3 days, wrapped in aluminum foil. Use frozen cauliflower florets, if you wish.

Makes: 4 servings
Active Time: 10 minutes
Total Time: 25 minutes

Canola or olive oil cooking spray

1 large egg

1 cup cooked and riced cauliflower*

1½ cups grated whole-milk mozzarella, divided

½ cup jarred no-sugar-added marinara sauce

3 cooked sausage links, thinly sliced

½ cup spinach, thinly sliced

Salt and freshly ground black pepper

1. Preheat the oven to 450°F. Mist an 8-inch-square dish with cooking spray.
2. Place egg in a large bowl and beat with a wire whisk until foamy. Add cauliflower and 1 cup mozzarella; stir well. Press cauliflower mixture evenly into pan.
3. Bake 10–12 minutes, until crust is golden and firm. Remove from oven and spread the marinara sauce over crust, then sprinkle with sausage, spinach, and remaining mozzarella. Season with salt and pepper.

* To rice cauliflower, cut into florets and steam 5–6 minutes over boiling water until fork tender. You'll need 1¼ cups florets to make 1 cup of riced cauliflower. Mash with a potato ricer or fork, or transfer to a food processor in batches and pulse to roughly chop. Cool completely before using in recipes. Riced cauliflower stores in the fridge, in an airtight container, for 4 days. Or freeze for up to 3 months.

4. Return pizza to oven and bake 2 more minutes, just until cheese is melted. Slice into 4 equal pieces and serve immediately.

PER SERVING: Net Carbs: 4 grams; Total Carbs: 5 grams; Fiber: 2 grams; Protein: 18 grams; Fat: 26 grams; Calories: 331; Foundation Vegetables Net Carbs: 3 grams

VARIATION

- Top pizza with ½ cup fresh mushrooms, drained marinated artichokes, roasted red peppers, or chopped olives.

Cheesy Chicken and Green Bean Skillet

If your family loves creamy casseroles but doesn't want to wait 45 minutes, this is your dish. Cheesy and rich, but quick and easy to make, this is comfort food at its best! To get dinner on the table faster, do the prep work the night before or earlier in the day—cut up the chicken, beans, mushrooms, and onions, and grate the cheese. Then store in sealed containers in the fridge until you're ready to prepare.

Makes: 4 servings
Active Time: 10 minutes
Total Time: 20 minutes

24 ounces raw chicken breast, cut into 2-inch chunks

½ teaspoon paprika

½ teaspoon garlic powder

2 tablespoons butter

2 cups green beans, cut into 1-inch pieces

1 8-ounce package mushrooms (button or cremini), thinly sliced

½ small red onion, minced

½ teaspoon salt

2 tablespoons coconut-flax flour blend

½ cup soy milk or chicken broth

1 cup grated Cheddar cheese

¼ teaspoon freshly ground black pepper

1. Place chicken chunks on a plate, sprinkle with paprika and garlic powder, and set aside.
2. Warm a large, deep skillet over medium heat. Add the butter, green beans, mushrooms, and onion. Sprinkle the vegetables with salt and cook 4 to 5 minutes, stirring occasionally, until the onion softens.
3. Add the chicken and the coconut-flax flour blend and cook 1 minute more, stirring to distribute the flour blend. Add the soy milk or chicken broth and cover. Reduce heat to low and simmer 1–2 minutes, until the chicken is cooked through.
4. Sprinkle the cheese over top of the chicken, season with pepper, and cover. Turn the heat off and leave on the burner for 1–2 minutes, until the cheese melts. Serve immediately.

PER SERVING: Net Carbs: 6 grams; Total Carbs: 8 grams; Fiber: 3 grams; Protein: 46 grams; Fat: 21 grams; Calories: 405; Foundation Vegetables Net Carbs: 4 grams

VARIATIONS

- In place of the coconut-flax flour blend, use ¼ cup finely ground flaxseed.
- Swap out green beans for broccoli florets.
- Top with ¼ cup chopped fresh basil.
- Phase 4: Serve over Atkins Cuisine Penne Pasta.

Asian Beef Stir-Fry

Take-out Chinese is convenient, but it can be full of hidden sugars. Instead, make this quick and easy version of a classic dish flavored with orange zest. Packaged beef strips are great time savers, as is jarred grated ginger. Like most Chinese food, leftovers can be reheated.

Makes: 4 servings
Active Time: 10 minutes
Total Time: 20 minutes

1½ pounds beef strips for stir-fry

2 teaspoons orange zest (or ¼ teaspoon orange extract)

1 tablespoon coconut-flax flour blend

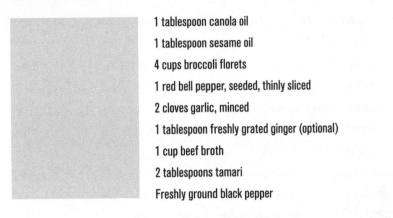

1 tablespoon canola oil

1 tablespoon sesame oil

4 cups broccoli florets

1 red bell pepper, seeded, thinly sliced

2 cloves garlic, minced

1 tablespoon freshly grated ginger (optional)

1 cup beef broth

2 tablespoons tamari

Freshly ground black pepper

1. Place beef on a plate and sprinkle with orange zest and coconut-flax flour blend. Heat a large, deep skillet over high heat. Add the canola oil and beef. Cook 2–3 minutes, stirring often, until the beef starts to brown. Transfer to a plate.

2. Reduce heat to medium. Add the sesame oil, broccoli, bell pepper, garlic, and ginger, if using. Cook 2–3 minutes, stirring often, until vegetables begin to soften. Return beef to the skillet along with broth and tamari. Cook 1 minute more, until the beef is cooked through. Season with black pepper and serve immediately.

PER SERVING: Net Carbs: 6 grams; Total Carbs: 10 grams; Fiber: 4 grams; Protein: 42 grams;

Fat: 22 grams; Calories: 408; Foundation Vegetables Net Carbs: 5 grams

VARIATIONS

- Omit the coconut-flax flour blend, but do not use all flaxseed.
- Replace the broccoli with snow peas or sliced asparagus. Or add canned water chestnuts or hearts of palm.
- Phases 3–4: Serve over brown rice.

Crockpot Pork and Salsa Verde ◑ ▤ sc

With 6 servings, this recipe is ideal for planned leftovers. Instead of wrapping the pork and sauce in lettuce leaf "tacos," you can also ladle it over the lettuce. Make up to 3 days ahead, cool completely, and refrigerate in an airtight container.

Makes: 6 (3-roll) servings
Active Time: 10 minutes
Total Time: 1 hour, 20 minutes

1 tablespoon canola oil

2 pounds boneless pork loin end roast

½ teaspoon mild chili powder

1½ cups jarred no-sugar-added salsa verde

1 lime, zested and juiced (or 2 tablespoons bottled lime juice)

18 butter or Bibb lettuce leaves

1 cup cherry tomatoes, chopped

1 cup finely shredded red cabbage

18 cilantro sprigs (optional)

Salt and freshly ground black pepper

1. Heat a large, deep skillet over high heat. Add oil and pork and sear for 3–4 minutes, without moving, until golden brown. Sprinkle with chili powder and turn over. Cook another 3–4 minutes, until the other side is golden brown.

2. Transfer to a crockpot and set to high. Add salsa verde and lime zest and juice. Cover and cook for 4 hours on high. Remove pork from crockpot and let it rest for about 5 minutes or until cool enough to handle. Shred with your fingers or two forks; return the meat to the crockpot.

3. Place about 2 tablespoons shredded meat and sauce into a lettuce leaf and top with 1 tablespoon tomatoes and 1 tablespoon cabbage. Roll up the package, top with a cilantro sprig, if using, and serve immediately.

PER SERVING: Net Carbs: 6 grams; Total Carbs: 8 grams; Fiber: 1 gram; Protein: 32 grams;
Fat: 9 grams; Calories: 250; Foundation Vegetables Net Carbs: 6 grams

VARIATIONS

- Replace the pork with an equal amount of chicken breast on the bone; decrease cooking time by an hour. Remove the bones and shred.
- Serve with a dollop of sour cream.
- Phases 2–4: Roll in a small low-carb tortilla.

Tilapia Patties on Baby Spinach

Love crab cakes but not the cost? Here's an inexpensive alternative. Mild tilapia takes well to seasoning and is palatable to those who aren't big fish fans. These patties can be made up to 5 hours ahead. Just form and coat the patties, then refrigerate—you can do the actual cooking when family or guests arrive. If you use frozen tilapia; just defrost in the fridge overnight before cooking.

Makes: 4 servings
Active Time: 15 minutes
Total Time: 40 minutes

6 cups baby spinach

3 tablespoon virgin olive oil, divided

1½ pounds fresh tilapia fillet

½ cup canola mayonnaise

2 tablespoons scallions, white and green tops, thinly sliced

2 tablespoons fresh parsley, chopped

2 teaspoons prepared Dijon mustard

½ teaspoon salt

¼ cup coconut-flax flour blend

2 tablespoons grated Parmesan cheese

1 lemon, quartered

1. Divide the spinach among four plates.
2. Heat a large, deep skillet over high heat and add 1 tablespoon olive oil. Reduce heat to medium and add the tilapia. Cover and cook

6–7 minutes, turning once or twice, until cooked through. Transfer to a large bowl to cool slightly.

3. Add the mayonnaise, scallions, parsley, mustard, and salt to the bowl. Fold all the ingredients together with a spatula until the mixture comes together in a sticky mass.

4. Shape the tilapia mixture into eight 4-inch-diameter patties. Place the coconut-flax flour blend and Parmesan on a plate or piece of wax paper. Mix with your fingertips. Coat the patties in the Parmesan–coconut-flax mixture and place on another piece of wax paper.

5. Wipe the skillet clean and add the remaining 2 tablespoons oil. Add the patties and cook 3–4 minutes. Turn and cook an additional 4 minutes. Transfer 2 patties to each plate beside the spinach and serve immediately with lemon wedges on the side.

PER SERVING: Net Carbs: 4 grams; Total Carbs: 9 grams; Fiber: 5 grams; Protein: 37 grams;

Fat: 38 grams; Calories: 517; Foundation Vegetables Net Carbs: 2 grams

VARIATIONS

- In place of the coconut-flax flour blend, use ¼ cup finely ground flaxseed.
- Swap salmon (including canned salmon), Pacific cod, or Artic char for the tilapia.
- Omit the baby spinach and serve over creamed spinach (see page 268).
- Serve with Lemon Tartar Sauce (page 265) instead of lemon wedges.

SAUCES

Lemon Tartar Sauce **7** ◑ ▤

Use this versatile sauce with chicken, fish, or pork. It also makes a tangy dip for crudités. Try it as a dressing drizzled on cooked or raw leafy greens, as well as cooked broccoli, green beans, or asparagus. Or use it instead of mayo in tuna or salmon salad.

Makes: 8 (2-tablespoon) servings
Active Time: 5 minutes
Total Time: 5 minutes

1 dill pickle spear, quartered

¾ cup canola mayonnaise

¼ cup grated Parmesan cheese

1 lemon, zested and juiced (or 2 tablespoons bottled lemon juice)

2 tablespoons heavy cream

½ teaspoon acceptable sweetener (optional)

1. Place the pickle in a food processor and pulse 10–15 times, until finely chopped. Add the mayonnaise, Parmesan, lemon zest and juice, cream, and sweetener, if using; process until smooth.
2. Serve immediately, or store in an airtight container, refrigerated, for up to 1 week.

PER SERVING: Net Carbs: 1 gram; Total Carbs: 1 gram; Fiber: 0 grams; Protein: 1 gram; Fat: 19 grams; Calories: 175; Foundation Vegetables Net Carbs: 0 grams

VARIATION

- Kick it up with 1 tablespoon pickled jalapeño or 1 teaspoon hot sauce.

Chipotle BBQ Sauce **7** ◑ ▤

Store-bought versions of this American favorite are usually packed with sugar in one form or another. This tempting, easy-to-make version uses sassy chipotle chile to jazz up chicken, pork, or beef.

Makes: 4 (heaping ¼-cup) servings
Active Time: 5 minutes
Total Time: 15 minutes

1 tablespoon butter

¼ small red onion, chopped

¼ teaspoon salt

1 cup diced canned tomatoes

1 tablespoon canned or jarred chipotle in adobo (see page 270), chopped

2 tablespoons red wine vinegar

1 tablespoon acceptable sweetener

1 teaspoon prepared Dijon mustard

1. Heat a small saucepan over medium heat and add the butter. Add the onion and salt and cook 3–4 minutes, stirring occasionally, until the onion has browned. Add the diced tomatoes, chipotle in adobo, vinegar, sweetener, and mustard. Cook 4–5 minutes, stirring occasionally, until mixture thickens.
2. Transfer to a blender and process until smooth. Serve immediately. Or store in an airtight container for a week in the fridge or in the freezer for up to 3 months,

PER SERVING: Net Carbs: 3 grams; Total Carbs: 4 grams; Fiber: 1 gram; Protein: 1 gram; Fat: 3 grams; Calories: 46; Foundation Vegetables Net Carbs: 2 grams

VARIATIONS

- Use apple cider vinegar in place of red wine vinegar.
- Replace the red onion with 4 cloves of garlic, thinly sliced.

Creamy Sweet Soy Sauce **7** ◖ ▤

This sweet but savory sauce lends itself to multiple uses. Brush it over roasted salmon, grilled chicken, or cooked shrimp, or toss with sautéed kale, bok choy, or broccoli. It's great with hard-boiled eggs too. Or brush it over skewered chicken cubes or raw shrimp along with vegetables such as Brussels sprouts, red and green bell pepper squares, and mushrooms before grilling. Finally, serve as a dip with raw vegetables.

Makes: 6 (2-tablespoon) servings
Active Time: 5 minutes
Total Time: 10 minutes

½ cup canola mayonnaise

2 tablespoons tamari

3 cloves garlic, minced

1 teaspoon freshly grated ginger

½ teaspoon acceptable sweetener

2 tablespoons chopped chives or scallions (optional)

1. Place the mayonnaise, tamari, garlic, 1 tablespoon water, ginger, sweetener, and chives, if using, in a large bowl and whisk well.
2. Serve immediately or keep in the fridge in an airtight container up to 5 days.

PER SERVING: Net Carbs: 1 gram; Total Carbs: 1 gram; Fiber: 0 grams; Protein: 1 gram; Fat: 15 grams; Calories: 140; Foundation Vegetables Net Carbs: 0 grams

VARIATION

- For crispy baked chicken, coat one side of a boneless, skinless chicken breast with 1 tablespoon Creamy Sweet Soy Sauce, then press chicken into coconut-flax flour blend. Bake at 350°F, uncovered and sauce side up, for 40 minutes.

Parmesan-Garlic White Sauce **7** ◐ ▤

Step aside, Alfredo, there's a new sauce in town! Use this sauce, which is thickened with coconut flour, to enrich your chicken, shrimp, and greens. Or wilt 4 cups baby spinach and top with ½ cup sauce for creamed spinach pronto. Sauté chicken cubes and chopped mushrooms with 1 tablespoon olive oil and top with this sauce for classic comfort food. Or top grilled or sautéed shrimp with it for a creamy version of shrimp scampi.

Makes: 6 (¼-cup) servings
Active Time: 10 minutes
Total Time: 5 minutes

1 tablespoon butter

4 cloves garlic, minced

2 tablespoon coconut flour (see page 249)

1 cup chicken broth

1 cup grated Parmesan cheese

½ cup heavy cream

¼ teaspoon salt

¼ teaspoon freshly ground pepper

2 tablespoons minced parsley

1. Heat a medium saucepan over medium heat. Add the butter and garlic and cook 2–3 minutes, stirring occasionally, until the garlic is fragrant. Add the coconut flour and cook 1 minute more, until the flour coats the garlic.
2. Slowly add the broth and whisk. Bring to a simmer, and then add the Parmesan and cream. Simmer 3–4 minutes, whisking occasionally, until the mixture forms a thick sauce. Sprinkle with salt, pepper, and parsley and serve immediately. It also reheats beautifully. Store in an airtight container, refrigerated, up to 1 week.

PER SERVING: Net Carbs: 2 grams; Total Carbs: 3 grams; Fiber: 1 gram; Protein: 6 grams;

Fat: 14 grams; Calories: 159; Foundation Vegetables Net Carbs: 0 grams

Speedy, Spicy, Chunky Tomato Sauce 🌓 🗄

This chunky sauce looks like traditional marinara layered with pepperoni. But it can also be given a creamy texture like vodka sauce. Marinara isn't just for pasta. It also makes a tasty topper for green veggies, particularly with a sprinkle of grated cheese.

Makes: 4 servings
Active Time: 10 minutes
Total Time: 30 minutes

1 tablespoon virgin olive oil

¼ cup chopped nitrate-free pepperoni

2 cloves garlic, thinly sliced

1 teaspoon red chile flakes

½ teaspoon salt

½ pound fresh tomatoes, chopped

1 sprig fresh basil

1. Warm a large skillet over medium high heat, add the olive oil, pepperoni, garlic, red chile flakes, and salt. Cook 1–2 minutes, until the garlic is fragrant. Add the tomatoes, ½ cup water, and basil.
2. Increase the heat to high and bring to a boil. Immediately decrease the heat to low and simmer 18–20 minutes, until a thick sauce forms. Serve immediately, or refrigerate in an airtight container up to 1 week.

PER SERVING: Net Carbs: 3 grams; Total Carbs: 3 grams; Fiber: 1 gram; Protein: 3 grams;

Fat: 7 grams; Calories: 85; Foundation Vegetables Net Carbs: 2 grams

VARIATIONS

- Use mild nitrate-free salami in place of pepperoni to dial down the heat.
- *Fast, Spicy, Smooth Tomato Sauce:* After Step 2, remove the basil sprig and puree the sauce in a blender. If desired, add 2 tablespoons vodka with the tomatoes and water.

MAIN DISH SALADS

Chipotle Shrimp Salad

Chipotle in adobo is smoked jalapeños marinated in a garlicky tomato sauce. Look for small jars or cans in the international aisle of your grocery store. Freeze leftovers in plastic sandwich bags. For less heat, remove the seeds or reduce the amount of chipotle. You can save significantly by buying whole shrimp. Remove the shells and veins under cold running water before cooking. Or to save time and fuss, purchase cooked shelled shrimp.

Makes: 4 servings
Active Time: 20 minutes
Total Time: 10 minutes

1 heaping tablespoon chipotle in adobo, chopped

1 lime, zested and juiced (or 2 tablespoons bottled lime juice)

1 tablespoon extra-virgin olive oil

1½ pounds shrimp, peeled and deveined

2 cups finely shredded red cabbage

1 cup finely shredded green cabbage

½ cup cilantro, chopped, plus extra for garnish

4 cups baby spinach

1 Hass avocado, peeled, seeded, and thinly sliced

2 tablespoons butter

1. Mix chipotle with the lime zest and olive oil in a large bowl. Reserve lime juice. Add shrimp; toss to coat. In a separate bowl, toss the red and green cabbage and the cilantro. Divide the spinach between 4 plates and top with cabbage mixture. Top with ¼ avocado each.
2. Heat a large skillet over medium high heat. Carefully add the shrimp mixture and cook 3–4 minutes, stirring often, until the shrimp turns pink and are cooked through. Turn off the heat and stir in reserved lime juice and butter. Divide the shrimp between the four plates and top with the cilantro. Serve immediately.

PER SERVING: Net Carbs: 7 grams; Total Carbs: 12 grams; Fiber: 5 grams; Protein: 25 grams;
Fat: 17 grams; Calories: 292; Foundation Vegetables Net Carbs: 5 grams

VARIATIONS

- Replace shrimp with cubed chicken breast, adding an additional 2 minutes to cooking time. Or use leftover grilled or poached chicken breast instead, reheating for a minute or two.
- Phases 2–4: Warm low-carb tortillas, spoon shrimp into them, and top with cabbage.

Grilled Chicken and Marinated Kale Salad **7** 🕐 🗄

Kale is a mild-tasting relative of cabbage, full of vitamins A, C, and K. It's usually cooked, but it's also great raw, especially after being marinated. Unlike other salads, kale doesn't get soggy or lose its flavor when stored in the fridge overnight, making it an excellent (and portable) leftover. Save time by using grilled chicken from a deli or salad bar.

Makes: 4 servings Active Time: 15 minutes Total Time: 3 hours 15 minutes	¼ pound wax beans, trimmed 8 ounces kale, stems and tough ribs removed, leaves roughly torn 1 tablespoon sesame or extra-virgin olive oil 1 tablespoon red wine vinegar ½ teaspoon salt, divided ½ cup green or black olives, sliced 4 boneless, skinless chicken breasts ¼ teaspoon freshly ground black pepper 1 tablespoon canola oil

1. Heat 1 inch of water in a medium saucepan fitted with a steamer basket over high heat. When the water boils, add beans and steam 4–5 minutes, until fork tender. Drain and transfer to a large bowl.

2. Add the kale, sesame or olive oil, vinegar, ¼ teaspoon salt, beans, and olives to the bowl and toss gently. Cover and let rest at room temperature or in the fridge for 3 hours to soften the kale.

3. Heat a large skillet over medium-high heat. Sprinkle the chicken with the remaining salt and pepper. Add the canola oil and chicken to the skillet. Reduce heat to medium; cook 5–6 minutes, without moving, until the chicken is well browned. Turn the chicken and cook 5–6 minutes more, until cooked through and no longer pink in the center. Transfer to a cutting board and let rest 5 minutes. Slice each chicken breast into 8 pieces.

4. To serve, divide the salad among 4 plates, top each with 8 chicken slices, and serve immediately.

PER SERVING: Net Carbs: 6 grams; Total Carbs: 9 grams; Fiber: 3 grams; Protein: 39 grams; Fat: 14 grams; Calories: 313; Foundation Vegetables Net Carbs: 6 grams

VARIATIONS

- Replace the grilled chicken with leftover flank steak (see page 275).
- Substitute green beans for wax beans.
- After two weeks in Induction, top with ¼ cup chopped walnuts, divided among the plates.

Buffalo Chicken Salad

No need to worry about the carbs in bar food when you make it at home. These boneless, unbreaded chicken "fingers" are drenched in a delectable buffalo sauce that rivals what's served at the local watering hole. The minute amount of coconut flour has minimal carb impact, and the generous portion of chicken fingers turns an appetizer into a main dish.

Makes: 4 servings
Active Time: 10 minutes
Total Time: 25 minutes

1 cup beef or chicken broth

2 tablespoons Tabasco or other hot sauce

1 tablespoon tomato paste

1 tablespoon coconut flour (see page 249)

1 tablespoon butter

6 cups baby spinach

½ cup diced roasted red pepper

1½ pounds chicken tenders

½ teaspoon garlic powder

½ teaspoon mild chili powder (optional)

1 tablespoon virgin olive oil

1. Prepare the buffalo sauce: In a small saucepan, stir together the broth, hot sauce, tomato paste, and coconut flour. Bring to a slow simmer and cook 5–6 minutes, until reduced to about 1 cup. Whisk in butter.
2. Toss the spinach and roasted red pepper in a large bowl. Divide the salad among 4 plates.
3. Sprinkle chicken with garlic powder and chili powder, if using.
4. Warm the olive oil in a large skillet. Add the chicken and cook 4–5 minutes, turning once, until both sides are browned. Reduce heat to low and carefully add the buffalo sauce. Transfer 6 tenders to each plate and serve immediately.

PER SERVING: Net Carbs: 5 grams; Total Carbs: 8 grams; Fiber: 3 grams; Protein: 41 grams; Fat: 8 grams; Calories: 252; Foundation Vegetables Net Carbs: 4 grams

VARIATIONS

- Substitute fingers of turkey breast for chicken.
- Replace baby spinach with romaine or thinly sliced kale (stems and tough ribs removed).
- If you like your chicken "atomic" hot, add ½ teaspoon ground cayenne pepper.

Turkey Enchilada Salad

This salad uses crisp veggies, just like the classic version, along with protein-rich turkey, but cuts the carbs.

Makes: 4 servings
Active Time: 10 minutes
Total Time: 20 minutes

1 pound turkey cutlets

1 teaspoon mild chili powder

½ teaspoon cumin

½ teaspoon salt

2 tablespoons canola oil

1 green bell pepper, diced

½ cup canned no-sugar-added enchilada sauce

3 large heads romaine, thinly sliced

1 cup grated Cheddar cheese

1. Sprinkle the cutlets with chili powder, cumin, and salt. Heat a large skillet over high heat. Add 1 tablespoon canola oil and cutlets. Cook 4–5 minutes, turning once or twice, until turkey is cooked through and no longer pink in the center. Transfer to a plate.
2. Reduce heat to medium and add remaining 1 tablespoon canola oil, and bell pepper. Cook 2–3 minutes, stirring often, until the vegetables start to soften. Reduce heat to low and add the enchilada sauce. Stir well, scraping up any bits that stick. Turn the heat off.
3. Divide the romaine among 4 plates. Thinly slice the turkey cutlets and divide them among the 4 plates. Top each plate with one-quarter of the green pepper mixture and sprinkle each plate with one-quarter of the cheese. Serve immediately.

PER SERVING: Net Carbs: 5 grams; Total Carbs: 10 grams; Fiber: 5 grams; Protein: 38 grams; Fat: 18 grams; Calories: 344; Foundation Vegetables Net Carbs: 5 grams

VARIATION

- Substitute shredded whole-milk mozzarella for the Cheddar.

Crisp Lettuce Wedge with Sliced Flank Steak

This steakhouse-inspired salad uses nutritious, crunchy romaine in lieu of classic iceberg lettuce. The recipe calls for 2 pounds of flank steak because this cut doesn't come much smaller, providing 1 pound of leftovers for another meal, perhaps to top Marinated Kale Salad (page 271) instead of grilled chicken, or creamed spinach (see page 268). Note that the nutritionals are based on only half the flank steak.

Makes: 4 servings
Active Time: 25 minutes
Total Time: 35 minutes

2 heads romaine

2 pounds flank steak

½ teaspoon no-sugar-added steak seasoning

1 tablespoon canola oil

¼ cup heavy cream

¼ cup red wine vinegar

1 tablespoon extra-virgin olive oil

1 teaspoon freshly ground black pepper

½ teaspoon garlic powder

¼ teaspoon salt

¼ cup crumbled blue cheese

1 red bell pepper, seeded, diced

½ small red onion, sliced

1. Cut each head of romaine into 4 even wedges. Remove the cores, rinse under cold running water, and wrap in paper towels or clean dish towels. Place in fridge while you prepare the steak. Sprinkle steak with the steak seasoning.
2. Heat a large skillet over high heat. Add the canola oil along with the steak. Reduce heat to medium and cook 7–8 minutes, without moving.

Turn the steak and cook 7–8 minutes more, again without moving. Transfer to a cutting board and let rest for 5 minutes.

3. Meanwhile, make the dressing: Place cream, vinegar, olive oil, black pepper, garlic powder, and salt in a medium bowl and whisk until smooth.

4. Place one-quarter of the romaine on each of four plates. Cut the steak in half, reserving half for another recipe (see page 271, variation). Thinly slice the remaining half and divide among the plates. Sprinkle 1 tablespoon blue cheese over each salad, followed by 3 tablespoons dressing. Sprinkle with the bell pepper and onion and serve immediately.

PER SERVING: Net Carbs: 4 grams; Total Carbs: 7 grams; Fiber: 3 grams; Protein: 28 grams;

Fat: 25 grams; Calories: 365; Foundation Vegetables Net Carbs: 3 grams

All-Season Caprese Salad with Prosciutto

Caprese salad calls for vine-ripened tomatoes, which are usually available only in late summer. This main dish version uses jarred roasted red peppers instead. You can also find them at any olive bar. Make this salad ahead, cover with plastic wrap, and chill before transporting to your next potluck. Serve with one of our delectable soups for a satisfying meal any time of year.

Makes: 4 servings
Active Time: 10 minutes
Total Time: 20 minutes

1 cup fresh parsley leaves

1 cup fresh basil leaves

4 tablespoons extra-virgin olive oil

4 cloves garlic, chopped

¼ teaspoon salt

8 slices prosciutto

24 spears asparagus

Canola or olive oil cooking spray

8 ounces whole-milk mozzarella

1 cup roasted red pepper

1. Place parsley, basil, olive oil, 4 tablespoons cold water, garlic, and salt in a mini food processor or blender. Process until smooth. Set aside.
2. Cut each prosciutto slice into 3 long strips, for a total of 24. Wrap each strip around an asparagus spear; prosciutto will adhere naturally.
3. Coat a large skillet with cooking spray. Place over high heat and add the prosciutto-wrapped asparagus. Cook 5–6 minutes, turning occasionally, until the prosciutto has browned. Remove from the heat.
4. Thinly slice the mozzarella and fan it out on a platter. Top with the red pepper and prosciutto-wrapped asparagus spears and drizzle with the parsley-basil dressing. Serve immediately.

PER SERVING: Net Carbs: 7 grams; Total Carbs: 12 grams; Fiber: 5 grams; Protein: 24 grams; Fat: 30 grams; Calories: 400; Foundation Vegetables Net Carbs: 5 carbs

VARIATION

- Replace the roasted red peppers with two sliced vine-ripened tomatoes.
- Replace prosciutto with another 4 ounces mozzarella for a vegetarian option.

SOUPS, CHOWDERS, AND CHILI

Cream of Broccoflower Soup **7** ◑

You'll need two heads of broccoflower, a hybrid of cauliflower and broccoli. If you can't find broccoflower, simply use one head of broccoli and one of cauliflower. If so, cut a few minutes of prep time by buying them as fresh or frozen florets. The gentle cooking process preserves the antioxidant power of these tasty cruciferous vegetables.

Makes: 4 servings Active Time: 15 minutes Total Time: 30 minutes	1 tablespoon canola oil 1 small red onion, sliced in rings ½ teaspoon salt ¼ teaspoon freshly ground black pepper 4 cups broccoflower florets ½ teaspoon curry powder (optional) 4 cups chicken broth ½ cup mascarpone cheese

1. Heat a large stockpot over high heat. Add the oil, onions, salt, and pepper. Immediately reduce heat to medium and cook 4–5 minutes, stirring occasionally, until the onions turn golden yellow. Add the broccoflower and curry powder, if using. Cook 1 minute more, stirring often, until curry powder becomes fragrant.

2. Add chicken broth, 1 cup at a time, and 1 cup water. Cover and cook 5–6 minutes, until vegetables are tender. Turn off the heat and add the mascarpone. Puree with an immersion blender until smooth, or transfer to a blender to puree. Serve immediately.

PER SERVING: Net Carbs: 4 grams; Total Carbs: 6 grams; Fiber: 2 grams; Protein: 7 grams; Fat: 30 grams; Calories: 313; Foundation Vegetables Net Carbs: 3 grams

VARIATION

- Use a combination of broccoli, Chinese cabbage, and/or asparagus instead of broccoflower.
- Substitute cream cheese, sour cream, or heavy cream for the mascarpone.

No-Bean Chicken Chili

This chili is pale in color, thanks to shredded chicken spiked with lime and cauliflower, but it has a big, bold flavor—no beans about it! Cooking the chicken with its skin and bones yields superior flavor and keeps the meat from drying out. Letting it rest in the broth finishes the cooking without toughening the meat, as boiling does. This dish freezes well, so feel free to double the recipe.

Makes: 4 servings
Active Time: 10 minutes
Total Time: 45 minutes

3 chicken breasts, with bones and skin

½ teaspoon mild chili powder

¼ teaspoon salt

1 tablespoon butter

½ small red onion, chopped

1 red bell pepper, chopped

1 cup cauliflower florets

4 cups chicken broth

2 limes, zested and juiced (or ¼ cup bottled lime juice)

½ cup sour cream

½ cup chopped cilantro

1. Sprinkle the chicken with chili powder and salt. Heat a large stockpot over medium-high heat and add the butter. Add the chicken, skin side down, and cook 3–4 minutes, until skin browns. Turn. Add the onion, bell pepper, and cauliflower. Cook 2–3 minutes more, stirring the vegetables around the chicken.

2. Add the chicken broth and bring to a simmer over medium heat. Cover and cook 10 minutes, then turn off the heat and let rest 30 minutes.

3. Remove chicken from the soup. Peel off and discard the skin. Shred the chicken and return it to the pot along with the lime zest and juice. Stir well. Top each bowl with a dollop of sour cream, sprinkle with cilantro, and serve immediately.

PER SERVING: Net Carbs: 5 grams; Total Carbs: 6 grams; Fiber: 1 gram; Protein: 24 grams;

Fat: 16 grams; Calories: 263; Foundation Vegetables Net Carbs: 3 grams

VARIATIONS

- Add 1 tablespoon pickled jalapeño or grated pepper Jack cheese per serving.
- Replace the cilantro with chopped parsley.
- Add color and extra heat by replacing the sour cream with no-sugar-added salsa.
- Phases 2–4: Add ½ cup canned, rinsed chickpeas.

Taco Soup 🌓 🗒

Beef, tomato, and chili powder, the very ingredients used to stuff a taco, are at the heart of this savory main-dish soup, which lends itself to numerous garnishes. Avoid stirring ground beef; instead, searing it gives the meat a bit of crust that helps it remain as chunks instead of turning into fine shreds that can dry out. You can double this recipe and freeze leftovers in single portions.

Makes: 4 (2-cup) servings	1 tablespoon canola oil
Active Time: 10 minutes	1 pound ground beef chuck
Total Time: 30 minutes	2 teaspoons mild or hot chili powder
	½ teaspoon ground cumin
	¼ teaspoon salt
	½ small red onion, diced

1 small jalapeño, seeded and diced (optional)

1 tablespoon canned chipotle in adobo, chopped

4 cups beef or chicken broth

½ cup canned diced tomatoes

1 cup cauliflower florets

1 cup thinly sliced kale, stems and tough ribs removed

½ cup pitted black olives, sliced

¼ teaspoon freshly ground black pepper

1. Heat a large stockpot over high heat. Add the oil and beef. Without stirring, sear for 2–3 minutes. Sprinkle chili powder, cumin, and salt over the beef, and stir once or twice. Add the onions, jalapeño, if using, and the chipotle in adobo and cook 2–3 minutes more, until beef has browned.

2. Lower the heat to medium-low and add the broth, diced tomatoes, and cauliflower florets; simmer 9–10 minutes. Add the kale and olives and cook 2–3 more minutes, until kale is soft. Season with pepper. Serve immediately.

PER SERVING: Net Carbs: 6 grams; Total Carbs: 8 grams; Fiber: 2 grams; Protein: 29 grams;

Fat: 19 grams; Calories: 317; Foundation Vegetables Net Carbs: 5 grams

VARIATIONS

- Replace ground chuck with ground turkey.
- Phases 1–4 garnishes: grated cheese, chopped green onions, pickled jalapeños, or sour cream.
- Phases 2–4 garnishes: cooked black or other beans, torn low-carb tortillas.
- Phases 3–4 garnishes: crumbled whole-grain tortilla chips.

Creamy Basil-Spinach Soup with Bacon Bits 🌓

This elegant, bright green soup is incredibly easy to make but will make you look like a four-star chef! Spinach is a nutritional powerhouse, and its mild flavor pairs well with smoky bacon. Serve with a salad for a complete meal.

Makes: 4 servings
Active Time: 15 minutes
Total Time: 10 minutes

8 slices bacon

1 tablespoon virgin olive oil

½ small red onion, chopped

4 cups chicken or beef broth

8 cups baby spinach (about 5 ounces)

2 cups fresh basil leaves, plus 4 sprigs for garnish

¼ teaspoon freshly ground black pepper

½ cup mascarpone

1. Put the bacon slices in a large cold skillet. Place over medium heat and cook 5–6 minutes, turning often, until crisp. Transfer to a plate covered with a paper towel to drain. Set aside.
2. Warm the olive oil in a large stockpot over medium heat. Add onion and cook 4–5 minutes, stirring often, until soft. Turn down the heat to low and add the broth. Add the spinach, basil, black pepper, and mascarpone. Puree using an immersion blender, or transfer to a blender and process until smooth.
3. Divide the soup into 4 bowls and crumble two bacon slices over each. Top each with a sprig of basil and serve immediately. Or refrigerate and serve chilled.

PER SERVING: Net Carbs: 4 grams; Total Carbs: 6 grams; Fiber: 2 grams; Protein: 13 grams;
Fat: 37 grams; Calories: 389; Foundation Vegetables Net Carbs: 3 grams

VARIATIONS

- Use watercress instead of baby spinach.
- Use two packages of defrosted frozen chopped spinach instead of baby spinach. Add before blending and cook for an additional minute.
- Use cream cheese, sour cream, or heavy cream instead of mascarpone.
- After two weeks in Induction, top with a handful of toasted walnuts and use vegetable broth instead of beef or chicken.

Salmon Mushroom Chowder

This creamy chowder will remind you of holidays at the seaside! Mushrooms replace the usual high-carb potatoes. A small amount of coconut flour thickens the broth with a minimum of carbs. Don't forget the seafood seasoning, which flavors this otherwise mild chowder. Your fishmonger may be willing to cut up the salmon for chowder. Buying sliced mushrooms will save you a few more precious minutes.

Makes: 4 servings
Active Time: 10 minutes
Total Time: 20 minutes

1 tablespoon butter

2 celery stalks, diced

8 ounces white or cremini button mushrooms

½ small red onion, minced

½ teaspoon Old Bay or other seafood seasoning

¼ teaspoon freshly ground black pepper

3 tablespoons coconut flour (see page 249)

2 cups chicken broth

16 ounces fresh salmon, cut in 1-inch cubes

½ cup heavy cream

1 cup grated Cheddar cheese

1 tablespoon chopped parsley

1. Heat the butter over medium-low heat. Add the celery, mushrooms, onion, seafood seasoning, and black pepper; cook, stirring, for 5–6 minutes, until celery is tender. Stir in the coconut flour until it coats the vegetables. Stir in chicken broth. Bring to a simmer over medium heat, stirring frequently.

2. Add the salmon and cook for 2–3 minutes, until the fish is cooked through but not overcooked. Add the cream and cheese and cook, stirring, until the cheese is melted and the soup just begins to bubble. Divide the soup into 4 bowls and garnish with parsley and serve immediately.

PER SERVING: Net Carbs: 6 grams; Total Carbs: 9 grams; Fiber: 3 grams; Protein: 34 grams;
Fat: 39 grams; Calories: 524: Foundation Vegetables Net Carbs: 3 grams

VARIATIONS

- Replace salmon with tilapia or Pacific cod. Decrease the cooking time by 1 minute after adding fish to the broth.
- Use canned salmon (remove the skin and bones) or vacuum-packed salmon instead of fresh salmon. Add it after the cream and cheese, and just heat through.

SNACKS

Mozzarella Sticks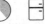

Gooey melted cheese inside a crunchy crust—what could be more irresistible? Here's another low-carb "renovation" of a typically high-carb
snack. Instead of breading, the sticks are coated in ground flaxseed.
Rao's Sensitive Formula Marinara Sauce is one acceptable sugar-free
product.

Makes: 6 (2-stick) servings	¼ cup ground flaxseed
Active Time: 10 minutes	¼ cup grated Parmesan cheese
Total Time: 1 hour	2 tablespoons finely chopped parsley
	1 teaspoon garlic powder
	½ teaspoon baking powder
	2 cups shredded whole-milk mozzarella
	1 cup riced cauliflower (see page 258)
	1 large egg
	Canola or olive oil cooking spray
	1 tablespoon canola or high-oleic safflower oil
	6 tablespoons no-sugar-added marinara sauce

1. Place the flaxseed, Parmesan, parsley, garlic powder, and baking powder on a sheet of wax paper. Mix with your fingertips or a spoon.
2. Place the mozzarella and riced cauliflower in a large bowl and mix
   well. Take 1 heaping tablespoon of the mixture and, using your fingers,
   form it into a 4-inch long stick. Place on a plate. Repeat with remaining
   cauliflower-cheese mixture. You should wind up with 12 sticks.
3. Place the egg in a shallow bowl and whisk.
4. Dip each stick in the egg mixture and then roll in the flaxseed-Parmesan
   mixture. Repeat, placing each on a freezer-safe plate. Cover with aluminum foil and freeze for 30 minutes (or more) to firm before frying.

5. When ready to serve, coat a large skillet with cooking spray and heat over high heat. Add the oil. Add the sticks and cook for a total of 4–5 minutes, turning once or twice and coating with another layer of the cooking spray. Serve immediately with hot marinara sauce.

PER SERVING: Net Carbs: 3 grams; Total Carbs: 5 grams; Fiber: 2 grams; Protein: 12 grams;

Fat: 14 grams; Calories: 195; Foundation Vegetables Net Carbs: 2 grams

VARIATIONS

- If the mozzarella sticks are completely frozen, preheat the oven to 400°F. Cook them according to the directions in Step 5, then slide the skillet into the oven and bake 5–6 minutes, until cooked through. Serve immediately.
- Replace the jarred marinara sauce with Fast, Spicy, Smooth Tomato Sauce (page 269).

Crunchy Asiago Crackers 7

These crackers rely on two kinds of cheese and ground flaxseed instead of grains. Aged Asiago cheese resembles Parmesan but is moister and milder. These crackers also make a great topping for most soups. Make the cracker batter up to 8 hours ahead and store in the fridge. Wrap leftover crackers in aluminum foil and keep at room temperature for up to 3 days.

Makes: 4 (5-cracker) servings
Active Time: 10 minutes
Total Time: 20 minutes

½ cup finely grated aged Asiago cheese

½ cup shredded whole-milk mozzarella cheese

¼ cup ground flaxseed

1 tablespoon finely chopped parsley

1 tablespoon sesame seeds (optional)

½ teaspoon garlic powder

½ teaspoon chili powder

Canola or olive oil cooking spray

1. Preheat oven to 400°F and place the rack in the middle. Cover a large baking sheet with parchment paper or aluminum foil.
2. Place the Asiago, mozzarella, flaxseed, parsley, sesame seeds, if using, garlic powder, and chili powder in a large bowl. Mix well with a spoon. (If the mixture seems too dry, add ½ teaspoon water.) Place 1 tablespoon of the mixture in your palm. Press into a disk and place on the baking sheet. Continue, making 20 disks and placing them 2 inches apart.
3. Coat the back of a spoon with cooking spray and press the crackers flat. Bake 8–9 minutes, until crisp and lightly browned. Transfer to a plate to cool. Serve immediately.

PER SERVING: Net Carbs: 1 gram; Total Carbs: 4 grams; Fiber: 0 grams; Protein: 8 grams;
Fat: 12 grams; Calories: 149; Foundation Vegetables Net Carbs: 0 grams

VARIATIONS

- Use Parmesan in place of Asiago cheese.
- Instead of sesame seeds, use 1 tablespoon finely chopped pumpkin seeds.

Crispy Kale Chips

A "superfood," kale turns up in salads, soups, and all sorts of other dishes. But who would have thought that kale could make a great low-carb stand-in for potato chips, popcorn, or pretzels? You can go to Whole Foods and spend a bundle for a little bag of these savory treats, or you make them yourself in a few minutes for a lot less money. Be sure to massage oil into the kale to make the chips crispy instead of greasy.

Makes: 4 servings
Active Time: 5 minutes
Total Time: 15 minutes

5 ounces curly kale, stems and tough ribs removed
2 teaspoons virgin olive oil
Pinch salt

2 tablespoons ground flaxseed

2 teaspoons sesame seeds

2 tablespoons grated Cheddar cheese

1. Preheat the oven to 400°F. Wash the kale, tear into 4-inch-wide pieces, and dry well with a paper or kitchen towel so that it will crisp better when baked.
2. Transfer to a large bowl along with the olive oil. Using your fingertips, rub the olive oil into the kale leaves until coated. Sprinkle with the salt, flaxseed, and sesame seeds. Spread the kale out on an ungreased baking sheet. Sprinkle evenly with the cheese and bake 10–12 minutes, until the kale is crisp and the cheese is melted.
3. Serve immediately. Or store in an airtight container at room temperature for up to 3 days.

PER SERVING: Net Carbs: 3 grams; Total Carbs: 5 grams; Fiber: 2 grams; Protein: 3 grams; Fat: 5 grams; Calories: 68; Foundation Vegetables Net Carbs: 3 grams

VARIATION

- Swap out the Cheddar for Parmesan cheese.

Zucchini Parmesan Fritters

These cheesy, herb-filled fritters would also work well topped with smoked salmon as part of a brunch menu.

Makes: 6 (2-fritter) servings

Active Time: 10 minutes

Total Time: 20 minutes

4 large eggs, separated

2 medium zucchini, trimmed and grated

½ cup grated Parmesan cheese

½ cup shredded whole-milk mozzarella cheese

¼ cup parsley, chopped

¼ cup fresh basil, chopped

¼ cup coconut-flax flour blend

½ teaspoon baking powder

⅛ teaspoon ground nutmeg

¼ teaspoon salt

Canola or olive oil cooking spray

3 teaspoons canola or virgin olive oil

1. Place the egg whites in a large mixing bowl. Using an electric mixer, beat on high speed until stiff peaks form. Set aside.
2. Place the egg yolks, zucchini, Parmesan, mozzarella, parsley, basil, coconut-flax flour blend, baking powder, nutmeg, and salt in another large bowl. Stir well until the zucchini is coated with flour. Using a rubber spatula, gently fold in egg whites until just combined. There will be streaks of egg white.
3. Coat a large skillet with cooking spray. Warm the skillet over medium high heat and add 1 teaspoon oil. Using a ¼-cup measure, pour out 4 fritters. Cook 2–3 minutes on each side, until lightly browned. Transfer to a plate. Repeat twice, using 1 teaspoon of oil and four ¼ measures of batter each time.
4. Serve immediately or refrigerate, covered in aluminum foil, and reheat when ready to serve.

PER SERVING: Net Carbs: 3 grams; Total Carbs: 5 grams; Fiber: 2 grams; Protein: 11 grams;

Fat: 11 grams; Calories: 159; Foundation Vegetables Net Carbs: 2 grams

VARIATION

- Use ¼ cup ground flaxseed instead of the coconut-flax flour blend.

Cocktail Shrimp with Lemony Garlic Sauce

If you use already cooked fresh or frozen shrimp, this new take on shrimp cocktail just requires assembly. If you purchase frozen shrimp, select medium or large ones. The small ones tend to get waterlogged and don't defrost as well. Make the dipping sauce early in the day and refrigerate.

Makes: 6 servings

Active Time: 5 minutes

Total Time: 10 minutes

1 lemon, zested and juiced (or 2 tablespoons bottled lemon juice)

¼ cup feta cheese

3 cloves garlic, minced

½ teaspoon prepared Dijon mustard

½ teaspoon Worcestershire sauce

2 tablespoons extra-virgin olive oil

1 teaspoon Tabasco or other hot sauce

¼ teaspoon salt

¼ teaspoon black pepper

16 ounces peeled and cooked fresh or defrosted shrimp

1. Place the lemon zest and juice, feta, garlic, mustard, Worcestershire sauce, olive oil, hot sauce, salt, pepper, and ¼ cup water in a blender or food processor. Process until smooth.
2. Serve each serving of shrimp with 2½ tablespoons sauce.

PER SERVING: Net Carbs: 3 grams; Total Carbs: 3 grams; Fiber: 0 grams; Protein: 18 grams;

Fat: 7 grams; Calories: 151; Foundation Vegetables Net Carbs: 0 grams

VARIATIONS

- Serve the sauce over leftover flank steak from the recipe for Crisp Lettuce Wedge with Sliced Flank Steak (page 275) or raw broccoli florets.
- Use the sauce as a dip for grilled or broiled skewered chicken, raw zucchini sticks, sliced bell peppers, and radishes. They'd make a great picnic treat.

DESERTS

Fudgy Pops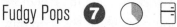

You may need to hide these from your kids! Better yet, make a double batch, but don't reveal the secret ingredient: spinach. The flavor is masked by cocoa. No ice pop molds handy? Use disposable small paper or plastic cups or even juice glasses, and insert a lightweight plastic spoon.

Makes: 4 servings
Active Time: 10 minutes
Total Time: 4 hours and 10 minutes

½ cup heavy cream

2 tablespoons unsweetened cocoa powder

½ teaspoon cinnamon (optional)

1 teaspoon vanilla extract

4 teaspoons acceptable sweetener

1 cup packed fresh baby spinach leaves

1. Place cream, cocoa powder, cinnamon, if using, vanilla, sweetener, spinach, and ¾ cup water in a blender and process until very smooth.
2. Pour into ice pop molds and freeze at least 4 hours before serving. To remove from the molds, run the molds under hot water for 30 seconds. Or simply leave the pops on the countertop for 30 minutes before serving to soften them enough for easy release.

PER SERVING: Net Carbs: 3 grams; Total Carbs: 4 grams; Fiber: 1 gram; Protein: 1 gram;
Fat: 12 grams; Calories: 118; Foundation Vegetables Net Carbs: 0 grams

VARIATIONS

- Instead of cinnamon, add ¼ teaspoon almond extract or a pinch of cayenne.
- Phases 2–4: Add ¼ cup bourbon or whiskey.

Devil's Food Panna Cotta **7** ◑ ▤

Italian for "cooked cream," panna cotta is a dessert made in heaven for Atkins followers. Be sure the water in which you place the gelatin is cold or the gelatin won't "bloom."

Makes: 4 servings
Active Time: 10 minutes
Total Time: 2 hours 10
   minutes

4 teaspoons unflavored gelatin

¾ cup half-and-half

2 tablespoons unsweetened cocoa powder

1 teaspoon acceptable sweetener

1 teaspoon instant coffee

1 teaspoon vanilla extract

1. Place four 3½-ounce ramekins on a large plate. Refrigerate while you prepare the panna cotta.
2. Place ¾ cup cold water in a small saucepan. Sprinkle with gelatin; let stand until gelatin has softened, about 5 minutes. Do not stir. Place over low heat and cook 1 minute, stirring well until the gelatin dissolves. Pour into a blender.
3. Add the half-and-half, cocoa powder, sweetener, coffee, and vanilla extract. Blend until smooth.
4. Pour mixture into chilled ramekins. Refrigerate on the plate until set, about 2 hours. Store up to 3 days, covered, in the fridge.

PER SERVING: Net Carbs: 3 grams; Total Carbs: 4 grams; Fiber: 1 gram; Protein: 4 grams;
Fat: 6 grams; Calories: 77; Foundation Vegetables Net Carbs: 0 grams

VARIATIONS

- Top with 1 tablespoon unsweetened whipped cream or drizzle with sugar-free chocolate or vanilla syrup.
- After two weeks in Phase 1: Top with 1 tablespoon toasted and chopped hazelnuts or walnuts.

Tiramisu Pudding 🥧 🗄

Our low-carb spin on this classic Italian dessert eliminates the lady-fingers but keeps the complex flavor. Be sure the soy milk–gelatin mixture is cool; otherwise the fat in the mascarpone will solidify and the pudding will separate. Torani and Walnut Acres make sugar-free chocolate syrup.

Makes: 4 servings
Active Time: 15 minutes
Total Time: 2 hours, 15 minutes

2 teaspoons instant coffee

1 tablespoon acceptable sweetener

8 teaspoons sugar-free chocolate syrup

1 cup plain unsweetened soy milk, divided

1 teaspoon unflavored gelatin

1 cup mascarpone cheese

1 teaspoon vanilla extract

½ teaspoon unsweetened cocoa powder

1. Place 2 teaspoons water in a small bowl with instant coffee and sweetener. Whisk well to combine. Stir in the chocolate syrup. Divide the mixture among 4 ramekins or parfait glasses.
2. Place ¼ cup soy milk in a small saucepan. Sprinkle with gelatin; let stand until gelatin has softened, about 5 minutes. Do not stir. Place over low heat and cook 1 minute, stirring well, until the gelatin dissolves.
3. Turn off the heat and stir in the sweetener. Cool soy-gelatin mixture 5 minutes or until it reaches room temperature. Whisk in the remaining soy milk, mascarpone cheese, and vanilla until smooth.
4. Divide the mascarpone mixture among the 4 glasses; the syrup mixture creates a swirl as you pour. Refrigerate, uncovered, for at least 2 hours. Sprinkle ⅛ teaspoon cocoa over each pudding and serve. Or store, covered, for up to 3 days in the fridge.

PER SERVING: Net Carbs: 3 grams; Total Carbs: 4 grams; Fiber: 1 gram; Protein: 7 grams;

Fat: 25 grams; Calories: 273; Foundation Vegetables Net Carbs: 0 grams

VARIATIONS

- Instead of refrigerating in ramekins, freeze the pudding mixture in ice pop molds.
- Instead of soy milk, use plain no-sugar-added almond milk or coconut milk beverage.
- Instead of sugar-free chocolate syrup, use hazelnut, caramel, or raspberry syrup.
- Top with shaved sugar-free dark chocolate.
- Phases 2–4: Stir in a few raspberries.

Lemon Crêpes

Crêpes use more liquid and eggs than pancakes do, making them thinner and less dense. Since the batter doesn't freeze well, make all the crêpes and keep leftovers for up to four days in the fridge.

Makes: 6 (2-crêpe) servings	4 large eggs, separated
Active Time: 15 minutes	¼ teaspoon salt
Total Time: 25 minutes	¾ cup plain unsweetened soy milk
	½ cup mascarpone cheese
	2 tablespoons butter, melted and cooled
	1 lemon, zested and juiced
	1 tablespoon acceptable sweetener
	1 teaspoon vanilla extract
	¼ cup coconut-flax flour blend
	2 tablespoons plain unsweetened protein powder
	1 teaspoon baking powder
	Canola or olive oil cooking spray
	3 teaspoons canola oil

1. Place the egg whites and salt in a large mixing bowl. Using an electric mixer, beat on high speed until stiff peaks form. Set aside.

2. Place the egg yolks, soy milk, mascarpone, butter, lemon juice and zest, sweetener, and vanilla in another large bowl. Whisk until well combined. Add the coconut-flax flour blend, protein powder, and baking powder. Add ¼ cup beaten egg whites. Using a rubber spatula, fold the dry ingredients and egg white into the mixture until just combined and a sticky mass forms. Add another ¼ cup egg whites and fold again until the mixture becomes lighter. Fold in the remaining egg mixture. Don't overmix; there will be small lumps.

3. Coat a large skillet with cooking spray. Place over high heat and add 1 teaspoon canola oil. Using a ¼-cup scoop, drop four scant scoops of batter onto the heated pan and spread out with the back of a spoon. Cook until the bottom is firm about 3–5 minutes. Flip and press lightly with the spatula. Cook another 1–2 minutes, until crêpes are cooked through. Transfer to a plate to cool. Repeat twice with remaining canola oil and crêpe batter. Serve immediately.

PER SERVING: Net Carbs: 2 grams; Total Carbs: 4 grams; Fiber: 2 grams; Protein: 11 grams;
Fat: 20 grams; Calories: 243; Foundation Vegetables Net Carbs: 0 grams

VARIATIONS

- Substitute ¼ cup finely ground flaxseed for the coconut-flax flour blend.
- Fill each crêpe with 1 tablespoon unsweetened whipped cream, with or without a splash of sugar-free flavored syrup or some grated sugar-free chocolate.
- Phases 2–4: Fill with fresh berries or 1 tablespoon no-sugar-added preserves. Or fill with whipped cream flavored with a bourbon or whiskey.

Green Tea Slushie **7** ◖

If you enjoy green tea ice cream, this slushie will become your new favorite. Target and Costco both sell green tea powder (also called matcha). Bigger supermarkets carry it in the international food section. You can also find it at Asian markets and natural food stores, or order it online. Double the recipe if you wish.

Makes: 2 servings
Active Time: 5 minutes
Total Time: 10 minutes

1 cup plain unsweetened soy milk

¼ cup heavy cream

2 cups ice cubes (about 8)

1 teaspoon acceptable sweetener

1 teaspoon vanilla extract

1 teaspoon green tea powder

1. Place all the ingredients in a blender and process until smooth.
2. Pour into two parfait or other tall glasses and serve immediately.

PER SERVING: Net Carbs: 3 grams; Total Carbs: 4 grams; Fiber: 1 gram; Protein: 4 grams;

Fat: 13 grams; Calories: 152; Foundation Vegetables Net Carbs: 0 grams

VARIATIONS

- Replace soy milk with plain unsweetened almond milk or coconut milk beverage.
- Add ¼ teaspoon mint extract and 1 tablespoon sugar-free chocolate chips.
- Replace the green tea powder with 1 teaspoon instant coffee.
- Serve with a drizzle of sugar-free chocolate syrup.

Afterword

Jeff S. Volek, Ph.D., R.D.

THE SCIENCE SUPPORTING ATKINS

I can virtually guarantee that you will be astonished when you hear about the current science supporting Atkins, especially the evolving new lines of research. The New Atkins Diet won't merely help you lose weight; in fact, that's just the tip of the iceberg. This chapter will provide a snapshot of the existing science supporting Atkins, as well as an overview of the emerging research on exciting new applications of a low-carbohydrate lifestyle. I have no doubt that after reading this chapter, you'll be confident that this is the best approach for lifelong health and wellness.

WHY ATKINS WORKS BETTER THAN OTHER APPROACHES

The number one reason the New Atkins Diet works so well is that it targets the fundamental problem most overweight people experience. That problem is insulin resistance. Simply put, if you have insulin resistance, and tens of millions of people in this country do, you don't metabolize dietary carbohydrate in an efficient way. Rather than burn carbohydrate for fuel, you tend to tuck it away as body fat. In fact, you are intolerant to sugars and starches. If you are carbohydrate intolerant, then it makes sense to limit sugars and starches; this is the cornerstone of the New Atkins Diet. When people who are carb intolerant follow Atkins, they experience amazing improvements in their health. Their metabolism shifts to burning mainly fat, which causes increased circulating levels of specific metabolites called ketones. Ketones are the preferred fuel for the brain and other tissues, and are being studied for a range of therapeutic applications. Running on a fat-burning metabolism is associated with higher energy levels, reduced carb cravings, higher satiety, and nearly effortless weight loss.

The science supporting Atkins goes back to at least the middle of the last century, but it has really picked up during the last decade. We now have a much better understanding of how and why controlling carbohydrates works to melt away fat and fend off diabetes, heart disease, cancer, and a host of other diseases.

WEIGHT-LOSS STUDIES

There have been a large number of studies comparing weight-loss responses between low-carbohydrate and low-fat diets, ranging from a few weeks to as long as two years. It's clear that, on average, following the Atkins Diet results in greater weight loss than other approaches higher in carbohydrate content. When you specifically look at those studies where the low-carb diet resembled Atkins and there was good compliance to the diet protocols, the results are nothing short of dramatic. For example, when my associates and I had forty overweight men and women consume either an Atkins-like diet or a low-fat diet for twelve weeks, the average weight loss was twice that on Atkins (22 pounds versus 11 pounds).[1] Weight loss varied significantly among participants, but the average loss for those on Atkins was greater than the loss by any single person on the low-fat diet. And when we X-rayed participants to determine body composition, we saw that those following Atkins had lost more total fat and specifically more belly fat.

Why does the Atkins Diet work so well for promoting weight and fat loss? This is still an open question among researchers, but the most likely reason is that restricting carbohydrates increases satiety, making it easier to restrict calories.

METABOLIC SYNDROME

Approximately one in ten adults in the United States has diabetes, and one in three has metabolic syndrome (prediabetes). A primary application of very low-carbohydrate diets in adults is to manage insulin-resistant conditions. Insulin resistance (carbohydrate intolerance) is the hallmark of type 2 diabetes and is also the primary defect underlying metabolic syndrome. Like other food intolerances, the most logical and effective approach to managing carbohydrate intolerance is to restrict the offending nutrient. To get right to the point, the Atkins Diet is a highly potent therapy for managing prediabetes and type 2 diabetes. In fact, it's many times more potent, and safer, than any medications for treating these conditions. Not only can the Atkins Diet prevent type 2 diabetes and slow down its progression, but it can also actually resolve all the signs and symptoms of the disease, in effect putting it into remission permanently.

What is the evidence for such powerful statements? First let's take an overview of the work on metabolic syndrome, and then we'll look at the key studies performed on individuals with type 2 diabetes.

Metabolic syndrome is best described as prediabetes and provides an early sign the body is struggling to manage dietary carbohydrate in a healthy way. The main features of metabolic syndrome are excessive belly fat; high blood levels of glucose, insulin, and triglycerides; low HDL cholesterol; and high blood pressure. You don't have to have all these signs, but if you have more than two, then you have metabolic syndrome. Studies estimate that approximately 64 million Americans have metabolic syndrome.[2]

You have metabolic syndrome if at least three of the following are present:

- Waist circumference: ≥ 40 inches (men) or ≥ 35 inches (women)
- Fasting triglycerides: ≥150 mg/dL
- HDL cholesterol: < 40 mg/dL (men) or < 50 mg/dL (women)
- Blood pressure: ≥ 130/85 mm Hg or use of hypertensive medication
- Fasting glucose: ≥ 100 mg/dL or use of hyperglycemia medication

The primary driver of metabolic syndrome is consumption of more sugars and starches than an individual can tolerate. A large number of studies have shown that the features of metabolic syndrome dramatically improve with carbohydrate restriction.[3] In fact, the Atkins Diet improves all the signs and symptoms of metabolic syndrome, often in dramatic fashion. Take, for example, the study in which my colleagues and I compared the Atkins Diet to a standard American diet in individuals with metabolic syndrome.[4] After three months, individuals in both groups lost weight, but weight loss and fat loss, including belly fat, were greater with the Atkins Diet. In the participants on the Atkins Diet, blood triglycerides plummeted by 51 percent, HDL ("good") cholesterol increased by 11 percent, and insulin sensitivity improved by 55 percent; there were even significant reductions in low-grade inflammation and functioning of blood vessels. This and many other studies clearly show the Atkins Diet is superior to low-fat/high-carbohydrate diets for managing metabolic syndrome.

TYPE 2 DIABETES

What if you have progressed past metabolic syndrome and have type 2 diabetes? The Atkins Diet could actually reverse your situation. Going back almost four decades, researchers have noted that type 2 diabetics consuming a very low-calorie carbohydrate-restricted diet experienced major weight loss (even as they retained muscle mass), saw improvements in blood cholesterol and blood pressure, and could discontinue their diabetic medication.[5]

Two decades later, an even more provocative study was published, showing that improvement in diabetes is more dependent on carb restriction than calorie restriction and weight loss.[6] Obese type 2 diabetics were fed two different diets, although both contained 650 calories a day, for three weeks. The two diets contained the same amount of protein but one consisted of 24 grams of carbohydrate per day, and the other 94 grams. The lower-carbohydrate diet resulted in significantly greater improvements in blood sugar control and sugar output by the liver. Interestingly, the magnitude of improvements was directly related to circulating ketone levels, indicating that the unique fat-burning state induced by the Atkins Diet specifically targets better diabetes management.

Ten years after that, it was shown that obese type 2 diabetics following the Induction Phase of the Atkins Diet (20 grams of carbohydrate per day) had remarkable improvements in plasma glucose and hemoglobin A1c, and a 75 percent increase in insulin sensitivity.[7] These extraordinary effects were observed after only two weeks on the diet. There are also studies of longer duration. After more than one year of consuming an Atkinslike diet, type 2 diabetics lost significant weight and had remarkable improvement in blood sugar (down 51 percent), total cholesterol (down 29 percent), HDL cholesterol (up 63 percent), LDL cholesterol (down 33 percent), and triglycerides (down 41 percent).[8] Other studies also support the long-term efficacy of the Atkins Diet in managing complications of type 2 diabetes.[9–11]

IMPROVED BLOOD LIPIDS

Blood lipids are the substances that transport fats (triglycerides and cholesterol) through your bloodstream. Elevated levels of these fats in your blood can indicate a higher risk for heart disease. The ones most commonly measured are triglycerides and total cholesterol, which includes two types: LDL cholesterol and HDL cholesterol. Extensive research has shown that the Atkins Diet dependably improves all these lipid markers, and therefore reduces your risk of heart disease.[12]

The most consistent response to restricting dietary carbohydrates is a decrease in circulating triglycerides. The effect can be quite potent, often slashing levels of triglycerides in half. After you eat a meal containing fat, blood triglycerides gradually increase and often stay elevated for several hours. The higher blood triglycerides go and the longer they stay elevated, the higher the risk for heart disease. After you have been on the Atkins Diet for several weeks, there is a dramatic improvement in your body's ability to process high-fat meals so fats don't accumulate in the blood.

As triglycerides plummet on the Atkins Diet, HDL usually increases. This is a positive response because HDL helps remove excess cholesterol from the body. The Atkins Diet does a better job at decreasing triglycerides while simultaneously increasing HDL than any other lifestyle factor, including exercise, and even outperforms most drugs.

In many cases, LDL will decrease or stay the same, but in some people it may increase. However, this variable response in LDL concentration from person to person is just part of the story. LDL particles come in different sizes, ranging from small to large. The Atkins Diet consistently decreases the smaller LDL particles. These are the more dangerous ones, as they are significantly associated with heart disease.[13, 14]

FATTY LIVER

The excess accumulation of fat in liver cells is tightly linked to overconsumption of carbohydrate, obesity, and insulin resistance (carbohydrate intolerance). Fatty liver significantly increases your risk of developing severe liver disease, diabetes, and heart disease. Fatty liver is not as simple to measure as BMI (body mass index) or blood cholesterol, and therefore statistics are not as precise, but it is estimated that between 20 million and 80 million Americans have this condition.

Similar to its effect on improving diabetes, studies indicate that the Atkins Diet has a profound benefit on fatty liver.[15, 16] In one provocative study, obese men and women with fatty liver were fed either a low-fat or a low-carbohydrate Atkins-like diet. The low-fat diet contained slightly fewer calories and significantly more carbohydrate (169 grams a day) compared to the Atkins Diet (26 grams a day). Fatty liver was measured using sophisticated imaging techniques. Despite being higher in calories, after just two weeks the Atkins Diet led to significantly greater reductions in liver fat content.[16] This demonstrates that the Atkins Diet is a more effective treatment for fatty liver independent of weight loss.

WHAT ABOUT SATURATED FATS?

At this point you might be concerned about whether eating saturated fat on the Atkins Diet will affect your health. Fortunately, that has been the focus of rigorous research, and the results may shock you. Remember, the basic concept of the Atkins Diet is to reduce dietary carbohydrates to the point that you are able to preferentially burn your stored body fat as well as the fat you eat. It turns out that when you are on the Atkins Diet your body prefers to burn saturated fat for fuel. That means that the saturated fat you eat does not accumulate in your arteries or on your hips. Instead, it is promptly burned as fuel. Two studies have shown that levels of saturated fat in the blood actually go down in individuals consuming the Atkins Diet, whether or not they lost weight.[17, 18] This is an important effect of the Atkins Diet because people with higher levels of saturated fat in their blood have an increased risk of developing metabolic syndrome,[19] diabetes,[20] heart attack,[21] and heart failure.[22] The bottom line is that there is no need to fear or avoid saturated fat on the Atkins Diet; in fact, it provides a preferred fuel, adds flavor to food, and promotes satiety.

You might also be interested to learn that researchers are seriously reevaluating the saturated fat paradigm. Large comprehensive reviews performed in recent years have all failed to find any association between saturated fat intake and incidence of heart disease.[23, 24]

EPILEPSY AND OTHER NEUROLOGICAL DISEASES

Very low-carbohydrate diets have long been known to be an effective treatment for seizures. In many cases, such a diet can cure the disease within weeks, even in patients who fail to respond to epilepsy drugs.[25, 26] It is one of the more remarkable clinical benefits associated with the Atkins Diet. For children who are prone to seizures and who do not respond to medications, the diet is nothing short of a miracle. Although the medical literature is full of studies trying to understand how a low-carbohydrate, high-fat diet improves seizure control, it remains uncertain how exactly it works. The potent and rapidly expanding use of the Atkins Diet for treatment of epilepsy has inspired physicians and researchers to also study the effects of the diet on autism, brain tumors, and plaque development associated with Alzheimer's disease. Clinical trials are also under way on the use of low-carbohydrate diets like Atkins on head trauma, stroke, Lou Gehrig's disease (ALS), and depression.

CANCER

Cancer is a mysterious and immensely complex disease, but emerging evidence links many types of cancer to the disturbed metabolic state observed in obesity. More specifically, the growth and progression of many cancers appear to be connected to higher intakes of carbohydrate and stimulation of insulin production. Since the Atkins Diet restricts carbohydrates and lowers insulin levels, often dramatically, it makes intuitive sense that it might be an effective treatment and preventative strategy for some, if not most, cancers. The metabolic state induced by the Atkins Diet, with low insulin and increased levels of ketones (the by-product of fat burning), has been linked to reduced tumor growth in animal studies of brain, prostate, colon, and breast cancer. Although the basic science looks promising, there have been few published human studies to date investigating the Atkins Diet on cancer progression. One recent pilot study in women with advanced breast cancer showed that the Atkins Diet stabilized and even decreased tumor glucose uptake.[27] There are, however, a growing number of case reports and pilot studies as well as several ongoing clinical trials, and the preliminary results that have been published or presented at conferences have been positive. Expect more comprehensive results soon as this relatively new application of the Atkins Diet gains traction.

THE NEXT FRONTIER

The science supporting Atkins for healthy weight loss is impressive, but equally exciting is the application in a number of other conditions. The Atkins Diet causes accelerated fat metabolism, which results in production of specific metabolites called ketones that are being studied in much greater detail as therapeutic agents. It turns out that when a person's (or an animal's) metabolism runs on these small molecules, there is a host of positive effects, including decreased oxidative stress and inflammatory markers and improved tolerance to stress. Besides the neurological diseases and cancers mentioned above, basic and applied scientists are studying the mechanisms of how this fat-burning state induced by the Atkins Diet improves wound healing, ameliorates post-traumatic stress disorder, slows down the aging process, and much more. Research is not just focused on weight loss and clinical applications. Recreational and elite athletes and soldiers are also using the Atkins Diet to enhance their physical and mental performance and speed recovery from exercise.

SUMMARY

There is already an impressive amount of research supporting the Atkins Diet for weight loss and metabolic health. The next decade will be enlightening as research continues to shed light on new applications. Because of the existing science and a long history of use, we can say with confidence that not only is the Atkins Diet safe, it's also a disease-fighting, health-promoting lifestyle.

▲ ▲ ▲

Dr. Volek is a professor in the number-one-ranked Department of Kinesiology at the University of Connecticut, where he teaches and leads a research team that explores the physiologic impact of various dietary and exercise regimens and nutritional supplements. Dr. Volek's most significant line of work has been a series of studies performed over the last fifteen years aimed at better understanding what constitutes a well-formulated low-carbohydrate diet and its impact on obesity, body composition, adaptations to training, and overall metabolic health. This line of work has shown profound effects of carbohydrate restriction on overall health and well-being, as well as on peak performance. He has published more than 250 scientific manuscripts and presented more than 100 talks at scientific and industry conferences in eight countries. Dr. Volek is coauthor of the *New York Times* bestselling *The New Atkins for a New You*, published in March 2010, and has subsequently self-published *The Art and Science of Low Carbohydrate Living* and *The Art and Science of Low Carbohydrate Performance*, which delve deeper into the science and application of low-carbohydrate diets.

Notes

1. J. S. Volek, S. D. Phinney, C. E. Forsythe, E. E. Quann, R. J. Wood, M. J. Puglisi, et al., "Carbohydrate Restriction Has a More Favorable Impact on the Metabolic Syndrome Than a Low Fat Diet," *Lipids* 44(4) (2009), 297–309.
2. A. Mozumdar and G. Liguori, "Persistent Increase of Prevalence of Metabolic Syndrome Among U.S. Adults: NHANES III to NHANES 1999–2006," *Diabetes Care* 34(1) (2011), 216–219.
3. J. S. Volek and R. D. Feinman, "Carbohydrate Restriction Improves the Features of Metabolic Syndrome. Metabolic Syndrome may be defined by the response to carbohydrate restriction," *Nutrition & Metabolism* (London) 2 (2005), 31.
4. J. S. Volek, S. D. Phinney, C. E. Forsythe, E. E. Quann, R. J. Wood, M. J. Puglisi, et al., "Carbohydrate Restriction Has a More Favorable Impact on the Metabolic Syndrome Than a Low Fat Diet," *Lipids* 44(4) (2009), 297–309.
5. B. R. Bistrian, G. L. Blackburn, J. P. Flatt, J. Sizer, N. S. Scrimshaw, and M. Sherman, "Nitrogen Metabolism and Insulin Requirements in Obese Diabetic Adults on a Protein-sparing Modified Fast," *Diabetes* 25(6) (1976), 494–504.

6. B. Gumbiner , J. A. Wendel , and M. P. McDermott, "Effects of Diet Composition and Ketosis on Glycemia During Very-Low-Energy-Diet Therapy in Obese Patients with Non-Insulin-Dependent Diabetes Mellitus," *American Journal of Clinical Nutrition* 63(1) (1996), 110–15.

7. G. Boden, K. Sargrad, C. Homko, M. Mozzoli, and T. P. Stein, "Effect of a Low-Carbohydrate Diet on Appetite, Blood Glucose Levels, and Insulin Resistance in Obese Patients with type 2 Diabetes," *Annals of Internal Medicine* 142 (2005), 403–411.

8. H. M. Dashti, N. S. Al-Zaid, T. C. Mathew, M. Al-Mousawi, H. Talib, S. K. Asfar, and A. I. Behbahani, "Long Term Effects of Ketogenic Diet in Obese Subjects with High Cholesterol Level," *Molecular and Cellular Biochemistry* 286 (2006), 1–9.

9. W. S. Yancy Jr., M. Foy, A. M. Chalecki, M. C. Vernon, and E. C. Westman, "A Low-Carbohydrate, Ketogenic Diet to Treat type 2 Diabetes," *Nutrition & Metabolism* (London) 2 (2005), 34.

10. J. V. Nielsen and E. A. Joensson, "Low-Carbohydrate Diet in type 2 Diabetes: Stable Improvement of Bodyweight and Glycemic Control During 44 Months Follow-Up," *Nutrition & Metabolism* (London) 5 (2008), 14.

11. T. A. Hussain, T. C. Mathew, A. A. Dashti, S. Asfar, N. Al-Zaid, and H. M. Dashti, "Effect of Low-Calorie Versus Low-Carbohydrate Ketogenic Diet in type 2 Diabetes," *Nutrition* 10 (2012), 1016–1021.

12. J. S. Volek, M. J. Sharman, and C. E. Forsythe, "Modification of Lipoproteins by Very Low-Carbohydrate Diets," *The Journal of Nutrition* 135 (2005), 1339–1342.

13. B. Lamarche, I. Lemieux, and J. P. Despres, "The Small, Dense LDL Phenotype and the Risk of Coronary Heart Disease: Epidemiology, Patho-Physiology and Therapeutic Aspects," *Diabetes & Metabolism* 1999; 25(3), 199–211.

14. K. El Harchaoui, et al., "Value of Low-Density Lipoprotein Particle Number and Size as Predictors of Coronary Artery Disease in Apparently Healthy Men and Women: the EPIC-Norfolk Prospective Population Study," *Journal of the American College of Cardiology* 49(5) (2007), 547–553.

15. D. Tendler, S. Lin, W. S. Yancy Jr., J. Mavropoulos , P. Sylvestre, D. C. Rockey, and E. C. Westman, "The Effect of a Low-Carbohydrate, Ketogenic Diet on Nonalcoholic Fatty Liver Disease: A Pilot Study," *Digestive Diseases and Sciences* 52(2) (2007): 589–93.

16. J. D. Browning, J. A. Baker, T. Rogers, J. Davis, S. Satapati, and S. C. Burgess, "Short-Term Weight Loss and Hepatic Triglyceride Reduction: Evidence of a Metabolic Advantage with Dietary Carbohydrate Restriction," *American Journal of Clinical Nutrition* 93(5) (2011), 1048–1052.

17. C. E. Forsythe, S. D. Phinney, M. L. Fernandez, E. E. Quann, R. J. Wood, D. M. Bibus, et. al., "Comparison of Low Fat and Low Carbohydrate Diets on Circulating Fatty Acid Composition and Markers of Inflammation," *Lipids* 43(1) (2008), 65–77.

18. C. E. Forsythe, S. D. Phinney, R. D. Feinman, B. M. Volk, D. Freidenreich, E. Quann, K. Ballard, M. J. Puglisi, C. M. Maresh, W. J. Kraemer, et al., "Limited Effect of Dietary Saturated Fat on Plasma Saturated Fat in the Context of a Low Carbohydrate Diet," *Lipids* 45(10) (2010), 947–962.

19. E. Warensjo, R. Riserus, and B. Vessby, "Fatty Acid Composition of Serum Lipids Predicts the Development of the Metabolic Syndrome in Men," *Diabetologia* 48(10) (2005), 1999–2005.

20. P. S. Patel, S. J. Sharp, E. Jansen, R. N. Luben, K. T. Khaw, N. J. Wareham, and N. G. Forouhi, "Fatty Acids Measured in Plasma and Erythrocyte-Membrane Phospholipids and Derived by Food-Frequency Questionnaire and the Risk of New-Onset type 2 Diabetes: A Pilot Study in the European Prospective Investigation into Cancer and Nutrition (EPIC)-Norfolk cohort," *American Journal of Clinical Nutrition* 92(5) (2010), 1214–1222.

21. L. Wang, A. R. Folsom, and J. H. Eckfeldt, "Plasma Fatty Acid Composition and Incidence of Coronary Heart Disease in Middle Aged Adults: The Atherosclerosis Risk in Communities (ARIC) Study," *Nutrition, Metabolism & Cardiovascular Diseases* 13(5) (2003), 256–266.

22. K. Yamagishi, H. Iso, H. Yatsuya, N. Tanabe, C. Date, S. Kikuchi, A. Yamamoto, Y. Inaba, and A. Tamakoshi, "Dietary Intake of Saturated Fatty Acids and Mortality from Cardiovascular Disease in Japanese:

The Japan Collaborative Cohort Study for Evaluation of Cancer Risk (JACC) Study," *American Journal of Clinical Nutrition* 92(4) (2010), 759–765.

23. M. U. Jakobsen, E. J. O'Reilly, B. L. Heitmann, M. A. Pereira, K. Balter, G. E. Fraser, U. Goldbourt, G. Hallmans, P. Knekt, S. Liu, et al., "Major Types of Dietary Fat and Risk of Coronary Heart Disease: A Pooled Analysis of 11 Cohort Studies," *American Journal of Clinical Nutrition* 89(5) (2009), 1425–1432.

24. P. W. Siri-Tarino, Q. Sun, F. B. Hu, and R. M. Krauss, "Meta-Analysis of Prospective Cohort Studies Evaluating the Association of Saturated Fat with Cardiovascular Disease," *American Journal of Clinical Nutrition* 91(3) (2010), 535–546.

25. E. H. Kossoff, and J. L. Dorward, "The Modified Atkins Diet," *Epilepsia* 49 Suppl 8 (2008), 37–41.

26. E. H. Kossoff et al., "Optimal Clinical Management of Children Receiving the Ketogenic Diet: Recommendations of the International Ketogenic Diet Study Group," *Epilepsia* 50(2) (2009), 304–317.

27. E. J. Fine, C. J. Segal-Isaacson, R. D. Feinman, S. Herszkopf, M. C. Romano, N. Tomuta, A. F. Bontempo, N. Negassa, and J. A. Sparano, "Targeting Insulin Inhibition as a Metabolic Therapy in Advanced Cancer: A Pilot Safety and Feasibility Dietary Trial in 10 Patients," *Nutrition* 28(10) (2012), 1028–1035.

Acknowledgments

Although my name is on the cover of this book, a project of this scope is always a team effort. I worked hand in glove with writer Olivia Bell Buehl, with whom I have collaborated many times. She takes my thoughts and words and polishes them until they gleam. Recipe developer Jennifer Iserloh, aka the Skinny Chef, created the quick and easy and Atkins-friendly recipes. Another Jennifer, Ms. Knollenberg, developed the meal plans and did the nutritional analysis of the recipes to ensure their compliance with the New Atkins Diet.

Literary agent Joy Tutela of the David Black Agency was with us all the way from the moment we began to ask ourselves the question: How can we bring a new generation of people into the Atkins fold by making the diet easier than ever to understand and follow? Consultant and strategist Marc E. Jaffe, who knows everything there is to know about the book publishing business, brought his wealth of experience and sharp mind to the project.

Colleagues at Atkins Nutritionals also played crucial roles as we refined the editorial concept. Chief marketing executive Scott Parker reviewed multiple iterations of the manuscript and regularly challenged us to simplify, simplify, and further simplify both the diet and the language describing it. He also suggested using visual components whenever possible. Brand manager Nicole Thompson performed the Herculean task of keeping the various components moving forward in sync, and on schedule, aided by assistant brand manager Carly Hofstedt. Nutritionist Vicki Cuce acted as my right hand, cheerfully researching and resolving countless questions and issues.

My good friend and associate Jeff S. Volek, Ph.D., R.D., one of the authors of *The New Atkins for a New You*, of which this book is an offshoot, wrote the chapter on the science attesting to the benefits of eating the low-carb way. Thank you, Jeff, for taking time away from your research on low-carb nutrition and fitness at the University of Connecticut.

Another shout-out goes to the nine Atkins followers who invited us into their lives and shared their amazing success stories. You are an inspiration to all of us who worked on this book and undoubtedly will equally inspire its readers.

Finally, thank you to our meticulous and insightful editor, Michelle Howry, and the rest of the editorial and production staff at Touchstone. With the publication of our fourth book, I can happily say that our working relationship is stronger than ever.

—Colette Heimowitz

Index

COMPLETE YOUR *NEW*
ATKINS LIBRARY
TODAY!